Working With Men

D1324301

One of feminism's key contributions to improving social work practice has been to expose the gender-blindness which has characterised social work policy and literature.

Working With Men is a controversial collection of essays written by feminists about men. In what has previously been an unexplored area of social work the contributors explore the issue of feminist work with men, highlighting the dilemmas which they have encountered in undertaking this work and concluding that feminist social work practice must include direct work with men as part of a broader strategy whose ultimate goal is the empowerment of women.

The book begins by acknowledging the contradictions inherent in feminism and identifies the experiences of the contributors and the assumptions which unite them. Following on from a discussion which explores the relationship between the growing literature on masculinities and developments in social work practice, each of the contributors describes her own experience of working with men. The range of subjects includes:

* social work practice with men in prison;
* youth work with boys;
* group work with men who have been perpetrators of domestic violence;
* divorce counselling with men;
* work with men on issues of sexuality.

The book concludes with an important discussion of the themes identified by the contributors, culminating in a Code of Practice for Feminist Work with Men.

Kate Cavanagh is Lecturer in Social Work at the University of Glasgow; **Viviene E. Cree** is Lecturer in Social Work at the University of Edinburgh.

The State of Welfare
Edited by Mary Langan

Nearly half a century after its post-war consolidation, the British welfare state is once again at the centre of political controversy. After a decade in which the role of the state in the provision of welfare was steadily reduced in favour of the private, voluntary and informal sectors, with relatively little public debate or resistance, the further extension of the new mixed economy of welfare in the spheres of health and education became a major political issue in the early 1990s. At the same time the impact of deepening recession has begun to expose some of the deficiencies of market forces in areas such as housing and income maintenance, where their role had expanded dramatically during the 1980s. *The State of Welfare* provides a forum for continuing the debate about the services we need in the 1990s.

Titles of related interest also in *The State of Welfare Series*

The Dynamics of British Health Policy
Stephen Harrison, David Hunter and Christopher Pollitt

Radical Social Work Today
Edited by Mary Langan and Phil Lee

Taking Child Abuse Seriously
The Violence Against Children Study Group

Ideologies of Welfare: From Dreams to Disillusion
John Clarke, Allan Cochrane and Carol Smart

Women, Oppression and Social Work
Edited by Mary Langan and Lesley Day

Managing Poverty: The Limits of Social Assistance
Carol Walker

The Eclipse of Council Housing
Ian Cole and Robert Furbey

Towards a Post-Fordist Welfare State?
Roger Burrows and Brian Loader

Working With Men

Feminism and social work

Edited by Kate Cavanagh and
Viviene E. Cree

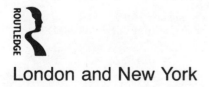

London and New York

First published 1996
by Routledge
11 New Fetter Lane, London EC4P 4EE

Simultaneously published in the USA and Canada
by Routledge
29 West 35th Street, New York, NY 10001

Phototypeset in Times by
Intype, London
Printed and bound in Great Britain by
TJ Press Ltd, Padstow, Cornwall

British Library Cataloguing in Publication Data
A catalogue record for this book is available from the British Library

Library of Congress Cataloguing in Publication Data
A catalogue record for this book is available from the Library of
Congress

ISBN 0–415–11184–6 (hbk)
ISBN 0–415–11185–4 (pbk)

If as evidence suggests men dominate an ideology that erases or ignores the significance of women and allows men to take for granted that their social constructions *are* reality, then transforming knowledge and ultimately patriarchy requires a challenge of that reality – even though it requires intruding where women are not always welcome.

(Scully 1990: 3)

Contents

Figure and tables

Contributors

Rowena Arshad is Lecturer in Equity and Rights, Moray House Institute of Education, Heriot-Watt University, Edinburgh. She is also Director of the Centre for Education for Racial Equality in Scotland, also based at Moray House Institute. Rowena's previous work experience was as Director of Edinburgh's Multicultural Education Centre and Education and Campaigns worker for Scottish Education and Action for Development, an agency linking Scottish and Third World issues. In addition to her current commitments at Moray House, Rowena is assisting Lothian Regional Council in the implementation of its Race Equality strategy. She has also completed a study of Central Regional Council's 'pre-five' provision in relation to black/ethnic minority uptake. She is writing and editing a multi-media pack on Anti-discriminatory Practice for students on teacher education courses. Finally, she is managing a funded project on 'Improving access onto social work, community education and teacher education courses for black/ethnic minority people' in collaboration with the Universities of Glasgow and Strathclyde; and preparing a 'redi-guide' of information on the position of black/ethnic minority people in education in Scotland. Of her many publications, most relevant to mention are: 'The Scottish Black Women's Group' in *Grit and Diamonds. Women in Scotland Making History 1980–1990*, by S. Henderson and A. MacKay (eds), Edinburgh: Stramullion, 1990; 'Alternative Vision', in *An Anthology of Women's Writing. Towards the Millennium*, Edinburgh: Polygon, 1991; 'Interconnections of Gender, Race and Class within Educational Contexts', in *Race, Class and Gender*, by S. Brown and S. Riddel (eds), Edinburgh: SCRE, 1992; 'Managing Equal Opportunities within Scottish Education Authorities. Lessons from "Race" ', in *Dia-

logue on Gender and Equality, by S. Erskine (ed), BERA, forthcoming.

Kate Cavanagh is a Lecturer in Social Work in the Department of Social Policy and Social Work at Glasgow University. Her particular research and teaching interests include domestic violence, child abuse, mental health and developing gender perspectives in social work. After graduating from the University of Stirling in the mid-1970s, Kate was engaged on a research project on domestic violence. She subsequently worked as an unqualified social worker before undertaking professional social work training at Warwick University. From 1981 until 1990, she practised as a social worker in a variety of contexts where she was actively involved in establishing services for women, before moving into social work education at Stirling University. From 1991 until 1994 she worked with Ruth Lewis and Russell and Rebecca Dobash on an evaluation of newly established programmes for perpetrators of domestic violence. She has written and published articles and papers on domestic violence and child abuse, the most recent being *Men's Programmes: A Research Evaluation*, Final Report presented to the Scottish Office and Home Office (forthcoming, 1995) with R. P. Dobash, R. E. Dobash and R. Lewis; 'Evaluating British and North American Approaches to Domestic Violence Interventions', in *Crime and Gender*, R. P. Dobash, R. E. Dobash and L. Noaks (eds) (1995) Cardiff: University of Wales Press, with R. E. Dobash, R. P. Dobash and R. Lewis. She is currently involved in the analysis of data gathered from the evaluation project.

Viviene E. Cree is a Lecturer in Social Work at the University of Edinburgh. Her specialist teaching areas include teaching on Sociology, Addictions, HIV/AIDS, and Sexuality. She also contributes to other course teaching on Skills and Foundations, and acts as a facilitator to student groups learning through the Enquiry and Action Learning method. She is Convener of Selection for the Master in Social Work course. Before coming to the University of Edinburgh in 1992, Viviene worked for sixteen years as a community worker, social worker and practice teacher in voluntary and statutory settings. She also undertook a PhD in Social Work, completed in 1992. The subject was a case-study of a voluntary social work agency in Scotland which had its roots in the nineteenth-century vigilance movement. Theoretical approaches drew on feminist theory and on the work of Michel Foucault. The thesis is entitled 'Social Work's Changing Task', University of Edinburgh, 1992. A book has been published arising out of this research: *From Public Streets to Private Lives*, Avebury, 1995. Viviene's current research interests centre on gender issues and caring. She is a member of the Lothian and Borders Gender Issues in Social Work Education Group. She is also developing new research around prostitution and young people.

Dorothy Degenhardt works at the University of Dundee Department of Social Work, where she is responsible for placement co-ordination and tutoring Diploma in Social Work students. Before joining the University of Dundee, Dorothy spent five years as a Lecturer in Social Work at Northern College of Education in Dundee, where her teaching included mental health, older people and community care, and gender issues. She also spent five years as a practice teacher. Dorothy's social work practice background is mainly in work with adults with mental health problems and with challenging behaviour in residential and community settings. Dorothy was involved in the setting up of Rape Crisis in Dundee, and ran groups for women with alcohol problems. She is currently undertaking a three-year distance learning course in person-centred counselling. She is also counselling adult survivors of sexual abuse in Central Region, working with a voluntary organisation, Open Secret.

Jane Forster works as Team Manager at the Naval Family Service based in Rosyth. The Naval Family Service offers an employment-based social work service for naval personnel, many of whom are men, and for their families. Jane's previous career in social work included working as a Tutor in the Department of Social Work at Moray House College of Education, and also as a family social worker at Barnardo's, and practice teacher at Family Care, an Edinburgh voluntary social work agency. Jane has a long standing interest in, and concern for issues around divorce. Her study *Take One Parent* was co-authored with Chris Stenhouse in 1980. A second publication, *Divorce Conciliation* (1982), was influential in the drive to establish a Conciliation Service for separating parents and their children in Scotland. Both studies were published by the Scottish Council for Single

Parents in Edinburgh. In 1988 Jane's new research resulted in another publication, *Divorce Advice and Counselling for Men*, an Occasional Paper from Scottish Marriage Counselling in Edinburgh.

Gilly Hainsworth is Project Co-ordinator at Pilton Youth Programme (PYP), a youth project for 12- to 18-year-olds based in a large council housing scheme on the outskirts of Edinburgh. PYP offers a variety of community-based services for young people, including group work, counselling and recreation. Before entering youth work proper, Gilly was a learning support teacher in secondary schools. She has also taught current affairs in a further education college. In addition to her current work commitments, Gilly is Director of Cranston Street Hostel for homeless women, and a management committee member of Edinburgh Streetwork Project, a project set up to help homeless young people in the city centre. Gilly's most recent research has been into the subject of young carers. She co-authored with Lami Mulvey and Aileen Mitchell a report entitled *Out of Sight* (1994), published in Edinburgh by the Scottish Education Department.

Jo Knox works as a social worker in the Social Work Unit at H.M. Prison, Edinburgh. ·In her social work practice she works extensively with perpetrators of sexual offences, who have been designated as a priority group for social work intervention. She is also an accredited practice teacher, and supervises social work placements within the prison. Jo leads teaching sequences on Criminal Justice on social work programmes at both the University of Edinburgh and Moray House Institute, and does Skills teaching at the University of Edinburgh, where she is also undertaking a part-time MSc course in Social Services Planning. Jo's present research interests lie in the question of risk assessment and sex offenders with learning disabilities. She has also been centrally involved in attempts within the prison to develop group work with long-term prisoners in relation to anger control.

Ruth Lewis holds a joint post at the University of Newcastle as a Lecturer in the Department of Social Policy and Relate Centre for Family Studies. Before taking up this post in 1994, Ruth was involved in research into crime, policing and drug use, and was Research Fellow at the University of Stirling, evaluating

Men's Programmes. She is currently a management committee member of Newcastle Women's Aid, and Sunderland Domestic Violence Forum. Her most recent publications include: *Men's Programmes: A Research Evaluation*, Final Report presented to the Scottish Office and Home Office (forthcoming, 1995) with R. P. Dobash, R. E. Dobash and K. Cavanagh; 'Evaluating British and North American approaches to domestic violence interventions', in *Crime and Gender*, R. P. Dobash, R. E. Dobash, and L. Noaks (eds) (1995), Cardiff: University of Wales Press, with R. E. Dobash, R. P. Dobash and K. Cavanagh; 'Measuring attitudes towards prisoners: a psychometric assessment', in *Criminal Justice and Behaviour*, 20 (2), June 1993, 190–8, with G. Ortet-Fabregat and J. Perez.

Siobhan Lloyd is the Head of the Counselling Service at the University of Aberdeen and a Lecturer in Sociology/Women's Studies. She worked as a planner and community worker before joining the Department of Social Work at the University of Aberdeen, where she was involved in social work education for eleven years. She co-authored with L. Hall *Surviving Child Sexual Abuse. A Handbook for Helping Women to Challenge their Past*, London: Falmer Press, 1993. This book is now in its second edition. Siobhan is and has been active as a campaigner against male violence towards women and children. She has run training courses on sexual abuse issues for a range of local and national agencies. She has also written and researched in this area, most recently in a co-authored Scottish study of specialist police units for the investigation of violent crime against women and children, entitled *Specialist Police Units in Scotland for the Investigation of Violence against Women and Children*, published in Edinburgh by the Scottish Office in 1993.

Monica Wilson is Joint Co-ordinator, CHANGE Project, University of Stirling. The CHANGE project was established in 1989 to develop a re-education programme based on criminal justice, for men convicted of violence towards their partners. Before taking up this post, Monica was a researcher for twelve years on a number of different subjects: marital violence; tenants' and residents' associations; housing for young single people; patient education. Monica has also taught part-time at both Napier University and Stirling University. In addition to direct work with men and their partners through CHANGE, Monica is heavily involved in training police, prison service, health service and social work departments in relation to men's violence to women, and contributes to seminars and conferences at a national and international level. Publications of most relevance to this book include: 'Battered wives: the victims speak' (1977–78), *Journal of Victimology*, with R. E. and R. P. Dobash and K. Cavanagh; 'Confronting domestic violence: an innovative criminal justice response in Scotland', in A. Duff, S. Marshall, R. E. Dobash and R. P. Dobash (eds) *Penal Theory and Practice: Tradition and Innovation in Criminal Justice*, Manchester: Manchester University Press, with D. Morran.

Cathie Wright is Co-ordinator/Trainer at Pilton Community Health Project's befriending scheme where her work entails training members of a post-natal support group to befriend other women. She also works as a freelance trainer in sexuality in the context of HIV/AIDS for workers in the caring professions, and is particularly interested in those working with people with learning disabilities. From 1981 to 1994 Cathie was a Senior Social Worker at the Edinburgh (now Lothian) Brook Advisory Centre, and co-ordinated Brook's education projects and an Urban Aid project in Craigmillar. Previous publications include: A. Frater and C. A. R. Wright (1986) *Coping with Abortion*, Edinburgh: Chambers; J. Burns and C. A. R. Wright (1993) *Sexuality in the Context of HIV/AIDS – a Trainer's Guide for People who Work with Young People*, Edinburgh: HMSO (currently reprinting). Cathie is working on a new publication on sexuality training for those who work with people with learning disabilities.

Series editor's preface

In the 1990s the perception of a crisis of welfare systems has become universal across the Western world. The coincidence of global economic slump and the ending of the Cold War has intensified pressures to reduce welfare spending at the same time that Western governments, traditional social institutions and political parties all face unprecedented problems of legitimacy. Given the importance of welfare policies in securing popular consent for existing regimes and in maintaining social stability, welfare budgets have in general proved remarkably resilient even in face of governments proclaiming the principles of austerity and self-reliance.

Yet the crisis of welfare has led to measures of reform and retrenchment which have provoked often bitter controversy in virtually every sphere, from hospitals and schools to social security benefits and personal social services. What is striking is the crumbling of the old structures and policies before any clear alternative has emerged. The general impression is one of exhaustion and confusion. There is a widespread sense that everything has been tried and has failed and that nobody is very clear about how to advance into an increasingly bleak future.

On both sides of the Atlantic, the agenda of free market anti-statism has provided the cutting edge for measures of privatisation. The result has been a substantial shift in the 'mixed economy' of welfare towards a more market-orientated approach. But it has not taken long for the defects of the market as a mechanism for social regulation to become apparent. Yet now that the inadequacy of the market in providing equitable or even efficient welfare services is exposed, where else is there to turn?

The *State of Welfare* series aims to provide a critical assessment of the policy implications of some of the wide social and economic changes of the 1990s. Globalisation, the emergence of post-industrial society, the transformation of work, demographic shifts and changes in gender roles and family structures all have major consequences for the patterns of welfare provision established half a century ago.

The demands of women and minority ethnic groups, as well as the voices of younger, older and disabled people and the influence of social movements concerned with issues of sexuality, gender and the environment must all be taken into account in the construction of a social policy for the new millennium.

Mary Langan
March 1995

Introduction

This is a book written by women about our work with men. Our aim is to redress the invisibility of men within social work literature and to describe some of the work at present being undertaken with men. In this process we hope to draw out an analysis of men in the social work discourse, an analysis which forefronts the complex and at times contradictory nature of men's power, as issues of class, race, ethnicity, disability and sexuality interconnect with and compete with issues of gender.

Our experiences of working with men are all different. Some of us have worked with male clients, colleagues and students in a mixed-sex setting. Others have turned our attention to men in single-sex settings, working with teenage boys, male offenders and violent men. Our paths into working with men have been varied too. Some of us have *chosen* to work with men, some of us have *had* to work with men, and some of us were *diverted* into work with men through our work with women. But in all these circumstances there remain common elements: different aspects of a common experience which we share. That shared experience is about confronting sexist structures and a male social construction of reality head-on, struggling to work within a social work system which is inevitably gendered and patriarchal in its foundations. This shared experience is the subject-matter of this book, as women from different work settings and different backgrounds describe their attempts to engage with and work with men in social work practice, social work education and social research.

THE SCOTTISH CONTEXT

The work we are describing is work which is taking place with men in Scotland. It is important therefore to give consideration to what we see as the Scottish context to our work. First, we must acknowledge that the legal framework of social work in Scotland is different from that of England and Wales (Social Work Scotland Act 1968). Criminal justice and probation are contained within the parameters of social work and local authority social workers supervise probation orders and work with offenders. One of the consequences of this is that it is much more likely that social workers in Scotland will work with men (Moore and Wood 1992).

Second, because of Scotland's relatively small population (around 5 million), the networks of feminists working in social work and social work education tend to be strong. Social work in Scotland, as will be discussed in future chapters, is overwhelmingly managed by men. Those of us who are feminists have found ourselves marginalised in our work, and there has been an urgent need to make links with other feminists, and to consolidate our position wherever possible. Thus many feminists are aware of the range of activities being undertaken by other women throughout the country.

This leads to a third, rather contradictory point. Scotland has played host to some very innovative and challenging projects centred on men. Domestic violence programmes aimed at changing men's violence to their partners began in the United Kingdom in Scotland. Likewise, Zero Tolerance first hit the streets and public arenas in Edinburgh before being transported to cities in England. In spite of, or perhaps because of Scotland's size and separateness, it has been possible to initiate creative and challenging work.

THE FEMINIST CONTEXT

We are all women who are prepared to describe ourselves as feminists, and central to each chapter is a description of how feminism has impacted on our professional and personal lives. It is important, however, to acknowledge that since feminism is a way of understanding and a way of being as well as a way of doing, the feminist perspectives which we bring reflect the sum total of our personal histories and class/race/ethnic/age positions. As our life experiences have been varied, so are our feminist standpoints. As a result, our understandings and interpretations of our work with men are different too. We make no apology for this. On the contrary, we believe that the diversity of women's lives, and the contradictory nature of women's oppression is such that a single feminist standpoint (Harding 1991) is not only unrealistic but also an unhelpful aspiration. Two definitions of the term 'feminism' take this discussion further. Gordon writes:

> I take feminism to refer to any body of thought that perceives women to be subordinated, perceives this subordination to be neither just nor immutable, and connects descriptions and analyses of women's conditions to hopes and plans for improving these conditions.

> (1991: 105)

Kelly, Burton and Regan propose:

> Feminism for us is both a theory and practice, a framework which informs our lives. Its purpose is to understand women's oppression in order that we might end it.

> (1994: 28)

There are two rather different but equally important points being made here. The differences between women are massive, and the notion of a category of 'woman' or of a single feminist standpoint cannot adequately express the reality of women's lives, and takes away from the contradictory nature of women's oppression (Ramazanoğlu 1989). But this does not mean that we do not have a common experience and a common goal to work towards.

What unites us in our work with men is the 'feminist lens' (Grant 1993: 109) with which we examine and interpret our experiences. Interpreting experience and offering analysis from that experience form the basis of our intellectual enterprise. Bringing together this collection has been a marvellous opportunity for all of us to think again about our lives and our work, and to discuss our feelings and ideas, some of which have been controversial and have made us feel uncomfortable. By facing up to the challenges in our work, we have been able to challenge the orthodoxy about working with men. This has been both a scary and exciting process.

But as Grant (1993: 181) argues, a feminist lens is not enough.

Feminism demands that critical examination and theoretical analyses are turned into action, and that we must always give attention to the liberation of women (Mitchell and Oakley 1986; Ramazanoğlu 1989; Langan and Day 1993). All the contributors have offered practical suggestions for future practice in working with men. But more than this, the book is based on a belief that if there is to be any improvement in the lives of women and children, men must change and women must be involved in setting the agenda here. Scully asserts that we must 'invade and critically examine the social constructions of men' (1990: 4). This should be the first step in our collective objective to change men.

In the tradition of feminist research (Du Bois 1983), we offer a broad summary of the assumptions which underpin our work with men:

- As society is sexist, so social work is inevitably sexist in its ideas and practices.
- Sexism is best understood as one oppression which connects with and at times competes with other oppressions based on race, ethnicity, class, age, disability or sexual orientation.
- There is no single category 'woman' and no single feminist standpoint. Nevertheless, women do share experiences of oppression based on gender, and feminists do share a common agenda based on reflection and a commitment to change (Lennon and Whitford 1994).
- As there is no single category 'woman', so there is no single category 'man'. Men are best understood in terms of masculinities (Segal 1990a; Brad and Kaufman 1994). This does not take away from their shared experience of privilege and power relative to women.
- Feminism must confront men and seek to change men: work with women is not enough.
- The so-called 'men's movement' should be discouraged from moving away from its roots in the women's liberation movement. Feminists must work with pro-feminist men to ensure that work with men remains women-centred in its practice and its goals.

AN OUTLINE OF THE CHAPTERS

The first chapter, 'Men, Masculinism and Social Work', written by Viviene E. Cree and Kate Cavanagh, sets the scene for the book, engaging with work which has already begun on feminism and social work and on men and masculinities. Viviene and Kate are critical of what they see as feminist social work's reluctance to debate the subject of men. At the same time they question much of the accepted wisdom which is emerging from the extensive and growing men's movement. They argue that feminist social work must address the issue of men: a refusal to do so may allow the expanding programme of 'men's work' within social work to proceed without a pro-feminist theoretical perspective and without an adequate understanding of women's experience. The negative implications this may have for social work and for women should not be overlooked or dismissed.

Jo Knox, in 'A Prison Perspective', presents a personal account of the dilemmas faced by women working with men in prison. In this chapter she vividly describes the setting in which she works – the drab, grey prison, with its overpowering sexism and macho attitudes. Then she goes on to offer a number of practical suggestions and observations about her work with men, and about how she has managed to survive and to challenge men in such a hostile environment. She urges a cautious but strong feminist response to working with men in prison.

Monica Wilson's chapter, 'Working with the CHANGE Men's Project', also describes work with violent men, but these men are in the community, at home with their partners and families, rather than locked up in prison. Monica charts the development of theoretical responses to domestic violence, and in particular, the development of a feminist perspective on domestic violence. She proceeds to examine the origins and the main features of the CHANGE programme, the first UK men's programme aimed at changing men's violent behaviour and attitudes towards their partners. Monica concludes with an analysis of the dilemmas she has experienced as a feminist working with men, and discusses the impact of the work on her as a woman.

In Chapter 4, 'Challenges in Working with Male Social Work Students', Siobhan Lloyd and Dorothy Degenhardt look at a very different subject: work with men in social work education. They begin their chapter with an acknowledgement that gender issues are now on the agenda in social work training. But they suggest that there is no theoretical framework for this work. Their chapter therefore sets out to provide that framework, drawing on key feminist themes including 'the personal is political', standpoint theory, a social constructionist perspective and an acceptance of the importance of theorising from experience. Siobhan and Dorothy go on to locate men in social work education and to make recommendations for training men in the future.

Viviene E. Cree's chapter, 'Why do Men Care?', pursues the question of men in social work education. Here she explores the personal histories and backgrounds of male student social workers in a research project about men in their first year of professional social work training. She argues that men's perceptions of social work and caring cannot be understood outside the context of the gendered assumptions and institutional practices within social work and within society. Viviene observes that men in social work training see themselves as different from other men, and value 'feminine' qualities more highly. However, their expectations of career advancement are also high, indicating that a more complex analysis is needed.

In Chapter 6, Kate Cavanagh and Ruth Lewis bring the subject back to violent men, but here their focus is on the theoretical considerations involved in doing feminist research with men as subjects and the many dilemmas which occur throughout the research process. In 'Interviewing Violent Men: Challenge or Compromise', Kate and Ruth describe their work as feminist researchers interviewing men convicted of violence against their partners. This research is part of a larger evaluative research project targeted at violent men and their partners. Kate and Ruth reflect on their work in terms of feminist research, and bring new insights to feminist research orthodoxy, including an analysis of 'challenge' and the concept of 'critical engagement'. This chapter widens the parameters of the debate around feminist research.

Jane Forster's chapter, 'Helping Men to Cope with Marital Breakdown', changes the tone and introduces a new area of discussion: men and counselling. Jane's subject is divorce, and more specifically, the effects of marital breakdown on men. She explores why men may be reluctant to seek counselling help and describes a pilot counselling project aimed at helping men (and therefore women and children) to cope with the aftermath of divorce. She also examines the challenges, dilemmas and implications for women social workers counselling men.

Cathie Wright in Chapter 8 picks up the subject of counselling, but this time examines counselling centred on sexual matters: pregnancy counselling and sexual problems counselling. 'Sexuality, Feminism and Work with Men' discusses the ways in which feminist ideas and practices have informed Cathie's counselling of men in individual and group settings around issues of sexuality. She notes that the advent of HIV and AIDS has brought with it significant changes in the context of her work.

In Chapter 9, 'Building Fragile Bridges: Educating for Change', Rowena Arshad tackles the complex area of race and gender, as she explores her work as a black woman training white men in anti-discriminatory practice. Rowena is critical of some of feminism's lack of attention to difference, particularly regarding race. She goes on to consider her experiences as a trainer and to describe a recently undertaken study which explores men's awareness of gender, sexism, and anti-sexism after undergoing anti-discriminatory practice training. She concludes that mixed-sex training seems to offer the best scope for challenging men's attitudes and behaviour.

Gilly Hainsworth's chapter, 'Working with Boys', discusses the feminist response to working with boys and young men. She provides a brief historical overview of the development of strategies in youth work, drawing attention to the current preferred practice position which involves women in work with girls, and men in work with boys. She argues that this is an unsatisfactory arrangement in feminist terms, because it denies young men the opportunities both to learn from and to relate to women, and it leaves many issues around power and oppression unchallenged. Gilly concludes with a case for women's continued involvement in work with boys.

The last chapter, 'Moving On', written by Kate Cavanagh and Viviene E. Cree, draws together the main themes from the book and considers the impact that writing the book has had on all the contributors. The book finishes with a suggested code of practice for feminist work with men.

Chapter 1

Men, masculinism and social work

Viviene E. Cree and Kate Cavanagh

The study of men is big business. Over the last few years, the two or three shelves devoted to women's studies in our bookshops have been transformed into good-sized sections on gender studies, with a whole new literature centred on men's psychology and socialisation, men in public and private life, and men's response to feminism. Men are now exploring their feelings, their friendships, their past and their future, their sexuality and their oppression: this new discourse owes much to the ideas and language created in the struggles of the women's movement (Canaan and Griffin 1990).

Men within social work have inevitably picked up and developed some of these ideas, and we can see the beginnings of a new agenda for men in social work in magazines such as *Working With Men* and research studies on men in traditionally female settings such as childcare (Ruxton 1992). But what has feminist social work had to say about men, as clients, colleagues and social work students? We argue that the feminist social work response to date has been to ignore the issue of social work with men and instead to concentrate ideological attention on social work with women. This book sets out to change this, to begin to look at the subject of social work with men from a feminist perspective.

FEMINIST SOCIAL WORK: THE CURRENT CONTEXT

Feminism has significantly influenced the theory and practice of social work in Britain. Feminist ideas have resulted in a systematic critique of social work at many levels, including its knowledge base, value system, use of language, ideology, organisational structures, modes of intervention and service provision.

Developments within social work education illustrate the changes which have taken place. The Diploma in Social Work gave social work permission for the first time to address issues of discrimination and oppression – 'to identify ideologies, structures and practices which are oppressive, and to change them' (Phillipson 1992: 8). The focus was on race, and other oppressions, for example, gender and disability tended to be combined, thereby seeming to be given a lesser priority. Nevertheless, in theory at least, the development of anti-sexist practice could potentially become a critical aspect of social work curricula. While the revised Diploma in Social Work seems likely to play down the significance of oppression, anti-disciminatory practice remains firmly on the agenda (Thompson 1993).[1]

One of the key contributions of feminism to social work has been to highlight the gender-blindness which has characterised social work policy and literature. Social work literature in the 1960s and 1970s was curiously non-specific in its targets of intervention, creating an impression that social workers were working with whole families, while in practice, social work remained an activity which provided services for a largely female population. Feminist ideas influenced and provided a critique of the 'radical' social work movement of the 1970s and 1980s (Bailey and Brake 1980; Langan and Lee 1989). Feminist social work theory has drawn attention to women's central position in the social work discourse as it has been formulated (Brook and Davis 1985; Hale 1984).

Feminist social work literature has explored different areas related to this central theme. Some writers have concentrated on recovering the historical origins of social work in women's philanthropic activity in the nineteenth century. Here the assertion is that social work has always been a woman's profession, and that man's arrival in social work has led to a defeminising of its activities and value-base. This has been explained as part of the professionalisation process – that men's participation in social work has coincided with social work's expansion and bureaucratisation. Women have been systematically excluded from the new positions of authority in social work (academic and work-based) as social work has become an increasingly attractive and high-status profession (Chafetz 1972; Brook and Davis 1985; Beagley 1986; Howe 1986).

There has also been a powerful critique of women in relation to the welfare state in general and social work in particular. Feminists have drawn attention to sexist attitudes implicit in social welfare policy and practice, and to the existence of powerful patriarchal structures which oppress women as service-users and service-deliverers (Wilson 1977 and 1980; Barrett 1980; Dale and Foster 1986; Pascall 1986). Much traditional social work practice has been based on unchallenged assumptions and negative stereotypes about women in their role as wives and mothers. Women are held to be responsible not only for their own lives, but also for those of their children, their partners and their dependent parents. Community care policy can be seen as part of the Conservative government's programme aimed at reducing state provision whilst making families (very often women) more responsible for the care of dependent relatives. Given this understanding, feminists have sought to establish more supportive and non-oppressive ways of meeting the needs of individuals and society (Walker 1982; Finch 1984).

Others have examined the differential treatment of women and men (girls and boys) in the statutory social work and criminal justice systems. Research has indicated that the sexual double-standard which assumes different rules of behaviour for women and men is still very much alive and influencing social work practice and decision-making today. Girls are still more likely to be removed from home because of their 'moral' well-being; women are still more likely to be imprisoned for lesser offences (Carlen 1983 and 1988; Gelsthorpe 1987; Hudson 1995).

At the same time as feminist social work theory has concentrated on putting women back on the social work agenda, feminist practitioners have devoted their attention to valuing and developing their work with women. Many social workers (including ourselves) who cut their feminist teeth in consciousness-raising groups in the 1970s began to look in the 1980s at ways of empowering the working-class women and girls with whom they were working. Current services were not adequately meeting the needs of our women clients who were pathologised and/or blamed. Some of us therefore turned to developing 'alternative' projects – women's groups, girls' groups and small-scale development projects around issues such as sexuality, violent partners and women's health. Some projects leaned towards the self-help, co-operative model of Women's Aid and Rape Crisis. Others were more therapeutic in style, developing feminist counselling methods (Chaplin 1988). Inevitably it has been more difficult to incorporate a 'woman-centred practice' (Hanmer and Statham 1988) into mainstream statutory services, but many women have done so, albeit with frustrating and exhausting implications for themselves. Feminist social workers working for the local authority have found themselves faced with an uphill struggle to have their work recognised and supported (Wise 1990).

MASCULINISM IN SOCIAL WORK

While feminism in social work has been struggling to achieve recognition, a new phenomenon in the form of the 'men's movement' has been developing. Masculinism has taken off in Britain and is today competing with and challenging feminist assumptions and ideas.

The men's movement in Britain was born in the late 1970s in response to the growing influence of the women's movement. Initially sympathetic to the oppression of women and acknowledging their part in that oppression, some men gathered in unusual conference with one another and, through a process of 'self-deconstruction', discussed the ways in which they oppressed women and explored the limits which patriarchy placed on the role of men (Tolson 1977). The early movement was essentially pro-feminist with supporters allying themselves to particular forms of oppression against women – for example, Men Against Violence Against Women; Men Against Sexism (Snodgrass 1977). While the motives of these men were laudable, the response by others to their position was met with no mean smattering of ridicule, incredulity and disbelief.

The late 1980s saw a rebirth of academic sociological interest in masculinity which continued to be largely pro-feminist (Hearn 1987; Chapman and Rutherford 1988; Brittan 1989). However, following publication of Robert Bly's *Iron John* in 1990 in the United States and 1991 in Britain, there has been a significant shift in the volume and content of literature on masculinity. A new masculinist literature has emerged to compete with pro-feminist ideas on masculinity: a new literature in which men extol traditional, patriarchal, hierarchical visions of 'true masculinity', and women are blamed for castrating men and for keeping men apart from one another. The new rallying cries are all about 'learning to get in touch with feelings', about 'finding your inner man', about 'bonding with other men' (Thomas 1993; Lyndon

1992) – bell hooks (1992) identifies that the most frightening aspect of the contemporary men's movement is the 'depoliticization of the struggle to end sexism and sexist oppression, and the replacing of that struggle with a focus of personal self-actualisation' (1992: 113)

But the new men's movement is more disquieting still. Not only does it not see itself as a response to feminism – as growing out of, and sharing a commitment to the aims of feminism – it is actively anti-feminist, and blames feminism for what it perceives as the demasculinisation of men. Faludi (1992), in her vivid account of the undeclared war against women, highlights the ways in which there has been a deliberate attempt to halt, and where possible to eradicate, the progress made by feminists on the hazardous road to equality. She regards the growing influence of the men's movement as part of an attempt to divide and isolate women at a critical point in their struggle for independence, equality and autonomy.

The impact of pro- and anti-feminist masculinist ideas in social work practice is growing. Historically the study of men had little place on the social work agenda. There have been some attempts by men to analyse men's place within social work's institutional structures (Walton 1975; Kadushin 1976; Howe 1986). Feminists have also shown consistent commitment to studying and drawing to public attention issues around male violence (Dobash and Dobash 1979; Hanmer and Maynard 1987; Scully 1990), around sexual abuse (Kelly 1988), around men's use of pornography (Dworkin 1981). But there has been little analysis of gender and men in relation to day-to-day social work practice. It is only in very recent years that a critique of men in social work has emerged, beginning with the publication in 1985 of Bowl's *Changing the Nature of Masculinity*, and illustrated by subsequent research which examines men in less stereotypically 'masculine' activities, such as caring for elderly dependants or working in childcare settings (Arber and Gilbert 1989; Ruxton 1992).

Today male social workers are increasingly involving themselves in, and dominating, social work with men. They are pressing for men-only activities – for example, men's groups and boys' groups – and masculinist themes (both pro- and anti-feminist) are beginning to appear in student social workers' essays and dissertations. There is in parallel with this a new rhetoric of 'men's rights' being rehearsed, as men assert their experiences of discrimination, witnessed in the congregation of men to fight the Child Support Act.

Unconnected with the men's movement, a new interest in men is emerging from government initiatives which promote new policies focusing on offending behaviour.[2] Cognitive behavioural approaches have become prominent as a means of intervening in work with male offenders. These perspectives, like those of the new men's movement, have been criticised for failing to address wider ethical, social and political issues (Sheldon 1995).

WORKING WITH MEN IN SOCIAL WORK

This is the world in which we, feminist practitioners and academics, find ourselves working. Feminism has rightly placed women at the centre of the social work agenda and has energised and encouraged women practitioners in their work with women. But at the same time, it has provided a rationale for opting out of work with male clients. The uncomfortable implications are that men's behaviour may have gone unchecked and that we may have played a part in reinforcing stereotypes about women's caring role within the family and within the social welfare net. Feminist explanations for not working with men may be expressed differently from conventional social work rationales for not doing so, but the outcome is the same – men's attitudes and behaviour towards women are left unchallenged.

In reality, in our private and professional lives, the great majority of us do relate to and work with men: only a very small percentage of social workers have no contact with men. Men are our bosses, our colleagues, our students and often our clients, notably if we are employed in criminal justice work, but also in community care and with children and families. This routine work with men has so far been unexplored in the feminist social work literature. Just as community care has been characterised as being principally about care by women, so social work has been said to be centred on work with women. The impact of this 'men-blindness' has been to leave a prominent area of social work unexplored and to diminish the complexity of the feminist analysis of gender in social work.

But there is another point at issue. In spite of a lack of feminist theoretical investigation of men in social work, increasing numbers of feminist social workers have chosen to work with men.

They have done so with the expressed intention of entering areas of practice which consciously set out to confront the nature of sexism at its source, that is, to change men's behaviour, as the contributors to this volume illustrate. This work has extended well beyond a consideration of incorporating feminist ideas about men into theoretical frames of reference. Scully reinforces this message. She argues that 'the de-bunking of patriarchy is not accomplished by focusing exclusively on the lives and experience of women' (1990: 3).

The outcome of the reluctance of feminist social work to address work with men has been that the feelings of isolation of women working with men have increased. We have found our-selves marginalised, challenged about our values, our beliefs and our feminism, by feminists and non-feminists alike. 'Real' femin-ists don't work with men. Fearing criticism and misunderstanding, we have been reluctant up to now to debate this taboo subject.

Whilst orthodox feminist social work has prioritised work with women, male social workers have been encouraged to take responsibility for their own and their clients' 'reconstruction'. This is another area of concern. How satisfied are we with the consequences of this work? Can we trust men to do this effec-tively? How can we evaluate this work if we have no part in it? These are important questions. The anti-feminist tone in much of the new masculinist literature warns against any complacency.

The feminist discourse around working with men must now be opened up. If feminism is about making judgements and acting upon them, about critical reflection and a programme of change, then it must extend its focus to practice with men. The absence of a feminist discourse around working with men leaves social work wide open to masculinist interpretations of the pro-feminist and anti-feminist variety, and whilst the latter is by far the more damaging to women, we must not assume that the former is to our advantage. The question is no longer 'do we work with men?' but 'how do we work with men?'

NOTES

1 The Central Council for Education and Training in Social Work's Paper 3 which revises the expectations for the Diploma in Social Work is less radical than its predecessor, Paper 30, in its acceptance of

ideas of oppression and anti-oppressive practice. It does, however, still contain a commiment to anti-discriminatory practice.
2 The National Objectives and Standards for Social Work in the Criminal Justice System prepared by the Scottish Office in 1991 require social workers to focus on offending behaviour.

Chapter 2

A prison perspective

Jo Knox

This chapter is a personal account of the dilemmas I have faced in working with men in prison, and an exploration of how I have sought to work with them. It does not set out to provide a definitive framework for social work in prisons. Feminist ideas and practices have added a new dimension to the arena of working with men, particularly in the field of sexual and physical violence towards children and women, creating a dynamic vehicle for intervention. I hope to contribute to this process by examining an area of work which social workers are increasingly recognising as a legitimate and appropriate focus for resources.

I do not believe that it is possible to work to a blueprint in social work. Each of us brings our own unique experience to the working relationship. For me, this involves being a woman and everything that has gone into creating the person that I am. This includes a developing awareness of feminist issues, in part a result of life experience, but also through an educational process. In this I believe I share common experience with other women. I do not share this commonality with men. Men develop their personae to a large extent *in relation* to women: they need to appear to be stronger, tougher, more able, more powerful. Chodorow (1978), in developing ideas about gender in relation to psychoanalytic theory, suggests that men achieve masculine identity through a rejection of qualities associated with their mother. Thus masculinity becomes a polarisation of feminine qualities (Newton 1994). I feel therefore that in this interplay women have a significant role in challenging men's perceptions of themselves.

My development to adulthood was undoubtedly influenced by having a mother as sole active parent. Her marriage breakdown and subsequent career achievement left me with a view that men were largely peripheral to life. Emerging at seventeen years of age from a girls-only school and this matriarchal background, I think I was oblivious to women's subordinate role in relation to men. Subsequent work experience made me conscious of the career limitations placed on women. Early in my working life, the realities of sexual violence and the victimisation which women experience in the court process impacted on me for the first time. Aged twenty and serving in the Women's Royal Air Force, I acted as 'professional friend' to a young woman who had experienced a serious sexual assault and attended the court martial of her attacker. I still remember with absolute clarity the feelings of anger engendered by the attempts of the defence, in an all-male court room, to justify the perpetrator's actions by blaming the victim's behaviour.

When I subsequently entered social work, an interest in the area of criminal justice led me to work with people who offend, without, I believe, considering that I would work almost exclusively with men. My gender awareness has developed over the years, most significantly through my experience of a traditional marriage and motherhood, which took me out of the world of work and independence and placed me in a situation where all my daily contacts were with women in a dependent, and relatively subordinate, role to men. Education and the challenge of other women has undoubtedly had a strong influence on me. My feminist perspective is essentially 'feeling'-based rather than an intellectually learned ideology. My awareness of feminist issues has developed in relation to my increasing consciousness of roles and relationships in both my personal and professional lives. I do believe that change is possible. I believe that men need to learn how the world looks through a feminist lens. I cannot see through a masculinist lens without a male conductor. I believe, therefore, that consciousness-raising for men demands an input from women.

THE PRISON CONTEXT

Since 1991, social work in Scottish prisons had been led by the National Objectives for Social Work in the Criminal Justice System[1] which focus attention on offending rather than welfare, and set out priority target groups. Perpetrators of sexual and physical abuse against children are the first priority, followed by other sex offenders, people with addiction problems, HIV and AIDS, and a range of those whose circumstances make them particularly vulnerable in prison – for example, people with learning disabilities or mental health problems. Within these priorities there is an inevitable tension between the managerial demand for offence-focused work and the client demand for welfare. This is compounded by the delicate balance of power involved in working within a secondary setting that has its own agenda and significant pressures. The social worker in this context strives to provide a service that is equitable with the professional task as well as meeting basic humanitarian need. The tension in this equation is one that is addressed to some extent (Moore and Wood 1992) but not as yet recognised at social work management level with the present emphasis on meeting National Standards. Prison-based social workers are left struggling with the conflict of failing to meet perceived need in order to meet directed priorities.

My work is in a large male prison accommodating around 700 inmates, with a prison staff of about 400. In all there are about thirty women in the organisation, including social workers, educators, clerks, prison officers and one female manager. The dominance of men in positions of power both confirms and perpetuates the traditional status and role of men in society, and in effect reinforces a situation that is increasingly challenged elsewhere. Given the relationship between crime and issues of masculinity it is worth considering the influence of such a male-dominated institution on recidivism. Prison social workers are employed by the Scottish Regional Social Work Departments although funded by the Scottish Office. Social work management, exclusively male, has to straddle an uncomfortable fence to satisfy these two organisational systems. In this rather awkward position the social worker endeavours to challenge offending behaviour whilst supporting and containing the anxieties that imprisonment engenders.

I work directly with men who have sexually and physically abused children, raped and abused adult women, murdered, assaulted, injured, robbed and defrauded. They may be serving anything from a few weeks to life imprisonment or be on remand awaiting trial. Within this context I shall examine the impact of the prison environment, and the effect that the regime and work has on me as a woman. I will also analyse the ways in which I engage with men in terms of intervention strategies, and explore some of the recurring themes in working both with and alongside men.

THE PRISON ENVIRONMENT

Previous experience of regularly visiting London prisons as a probation officer did not prepare me for the onslaught on my senses of becoming an 'insider' in a men's prison. Nor had previous contact with uniformed services prepared me for working with uniformed prison staff. My early weeks at the prison were traumatic. As an outside agent, business is conducted primarily with clients, and perceptions are based to some degree on what the client relates. However, when the prison is your place of work, there is a degree to which you share the experience and pain of imprisonment with your clients. The social worker becomes dependent in many ways on the prison officers; work is predominantly within the institution; and routines are prescribed to a marked degree by the routine of the prison. Social workers are daily subject to the physical conditions in terms of noise, smell, drabness – in fact to the sensory deprivation of imprisonment, where offices have no windows, and where interview rooms are basically cells. The prison key takes on particular significance. Without one it is impossible to move about freely from one place to another. The impact of the dark navy prison uniform is intimidating, and undoubtedly makes the officers seem larger than they appear in civilian clothing. (Interestingly, the women officers wear a much lighter shade of blue.) The uniform conveys authority. It is necessary to engage with this authority in order to enter and exit the prison, and for me this was a regular challenge for some considerable time. Without a uniform, social workers do not belong to the controlling regime and therefore have continually to reaffirm both status and role.

I feel it is important to retain these early images because they are experienced in a more extreme way by prisoners and this cannot be ignored in any determination to focus on offending behaviour. Work with men in prison involves helping them to adjust to, and come to terms with the totality of the deprivation which is the reality of their experience. This issue can often be the overriding one for the client, and needs a sympathetic and sensitive response which at the same time does not preclude other work taking place. The influence of the environment and the regime is so powerful that it can deflect from the impact of meeting men convicted of serious crimes. This clouding of issues is compounded by the social workers' welfare role, which operates on the principle that client need should take priority over work associated with the offence.

The physical aspects of the environment do, I believe, have an impact regardless of gender. This is reflected to some extent in the essence of machismo that appears to enhance the self-perception of many male officers and is also a significant issue for male offenders. Thus it appears to be important to be perceived as 'manly' – wearing shirt sleeves when the weather is freezing, for example. The presence of 'caring' social workers, male or female, is couched in confusion in an institution characterised by authority, control and containment. The tension in relation to caring and control is being increasingly challenged as the remit of the prison officer is developing to include welfare functions (SWSG & SHHD 1989).

Prisoners and staff alike share stereotypical views of gender roles. A woman entering a hall is immediately the object of surveillance. She may be watched silently by those in the vicinity, or subjected to some form of harassment by way of a whistle or some suggestive remark. Either way she is conscious of entering a male domain. Despite legitimate reasons for being there, she is an intruder. This can be exacerbated by staff who may choose to ignore her presence for a short time, encouraging her feelings of exposure. The washing facilities, including the urinals, are open areas in the halls and are impossible to avoid. Since 1992, with the increase in female prison officers on the halls, these areas have had minimal screening. Nevertheless, as a woman, when I enter a hall I feel conscious of invading male privacy and have developed a very fast walk whilst I examine intently any piece of paper in my hand if I have to pass these areas.

DISCRIMINATION WITHIN PRISONS

Prison portrays in a concentrated form a wide range of discriminatory attitudes. It may be that these attitudes are exacerbated by the discriminatory nature of imprisonment itself, or it may be that prison presents a microcosm of the outside social order. Social workers, especially women, are the recipients of a greater proportion of such attitudes and behaviours. In the context of this chapter I will focus on sexism, whilst acknowledging that many other forms of discriminatory attitude and behaviour cause distress within the prison. What is of particular concern is the endemic attitude about women's place in the world and how this is reflected in the demands made by prisoners on their families, how it impacts on offending behaviour in general as well as in terms of sexual offences, and also how men see their maleness in relation to their view of women.

A woman working within a male institution can be subjected to many forms of discriminatory behaviour. Such harassment includes wolf-whistles and the irritating male banter which frequently seems a necessary forerunner to any business discussion. Sexist remarks made by officers may also inhibit a female social worker's ability to carry out her tasks. For example, a student with whom I was working felt unable to obtain equipment needed for a group because of the sexist comments made by the keeper of the equipment each time she went to collect it. As a practice teacher, I am necessarily involved with issues like this in relation to students who are inevitably more vulnerable because of their status as learners and their unfamiliarity with the institution. Students and I work together to find strategies for coping with the difficulties as well as confronting inappropriate behaviour. It is helpful to recognise that the war against sexism is not going to be won by single-handedly challenging every situation that occurs within such an all-male environment, as these incidents can arise repeatedly throughout the day. There is a need to be aware of occasions where your challenge will be heard even if not accepted and maintain your energy for this. However, this approach is not unproblematic, and women may feel that they have compromised their beliefs by colluding with the male ethos and thus failing women. Neither is a confrontational approach necessarily helpful. Women in this working environment consequently need to develop a range of skills which will allow them to maintain their integrity whilst not impinging on their ability to carry out their task. Above all, a continuing awareness of these issues is required.

Some coping strategies which have been effective for me in situations of either direct or potential harassment and discrimination include:

• Simple unemotional and direct disagreement with sexist statements.

- Facial expression which denotes disapproval, particularly with men who have some awareness of the issues.
- Ignoring completely any sexual remarks or noises which you cannot directly respond to – for example, a wolf-whistle or similar noise emanating from some distance away, source unknown.
- Avoidance of eye contact at times when faced with a large group of unknown men.
- Modulation of responses, by being extremely cool to inappropriate remarks but responding normally or even warmly when treated androgynously.
- Being aware of the appropriate complaints procedure should such inappropriate behaviour persist.

What becomes evident in working in a large, male-dominated organisation is the difference between group and individual male behaviour. The most sexually harassing situations often occur when a woman is alone with a group of men. For example, a young women student subjected to a particularly offensive chant by a group of prisoners rightly felt that it was expedient not to challenge this behaviour. Issues of safety, confidence and support are important in deciding if and when to respond to these situations. Whereas on an individual basis men may show sensitivity towards women, a group may have an identity of its own and group members are often more likely to react in extreme ways towards women. It is a rare man who stands out against his fellows. Inevitably, one of the central issues at stake is power. Women working within this seemingly tough male bastion appear to threaten the status of staff and prisoners alike, each of whom has their own definition of the boundaries of their masculinity.

ISSUES AND STRATEGIES IN INTERVENTION

The prison-based social worker brings little in the way of material resources to her or his work, and is largely reliant on self and the skills and strategies of intervention that have been developed. Cognitive-behavioural approaches are the focus of much of the current literature in relation to offenders in general and particularly to sex offenders, and appear to offer the most promising prospects for intervention (McGuire and Priestley 1985; Ross et al. 1986; Marshall and Barbaree 1990; Dobash et al. 1993). Much intervention with sex offenders targets denial and minimisation, sexual knowledge, behaviours and interests, cognitive distortions about the offending behaviour, victim awareness, social functioning and relapse prevention.

I will now go on to explore my work primarily in relation to sex offenders, although many issues will have relevance for women working with other male offenders. The textbooks (Salter 1988; Marshall *et al.* 1990) describe particular approaches but seldom discuss the problems of actual practice. In examining intervention strategies, what is striking is the extent to which the issues which I must tackle with clients – for example, control, empathy, gender awareness and grooming – all have relevance and are mirrored in my work with men more generally.

Clarity about role

An essential ingredient of any successful intervention is clarity about role and purpose. A sense of caring is not exclusive to women (Lewis and O'Brian 1987; Arber and Gilbert 1989). People under stress can evoke feelings of compassion in either sex. However, as a woman striving to challenge male perceptions it is not helpful to adopt the maternal role as this reinforces stereotypical views about women. Thus, from the outset, it is necessary for a woman to be supportive and to convey a sense of concern about the individual but not to the extent that either the worker or the client forgets who the victim is and the task to be accomplished. There is a constant tension about who the real focus of attention is: the client, his past victim or the potential future victim. The fact that prison itself often victimises inmates creates an even more complex situation. An inmate I worked with who had sexually abused boys told me that a group of men had entered his cell and taken it in turns to rape him. Whilst this provided an opportunity to look at the impact of sexual abuse on his victims, the immediate aftermath of the crisis placed this man in the role of victim.

Imprisonment can create frequent crises for individuals. Although at times this can be a means of avoiding agreed work it can also produce a disequilibrium in the individual which makes them more open to being helped (Golan 1978). It was shortly after this incident that my client moved forward considerably in describing his previous life style, which was highly relevant to his offending behaviour. This example illustrates the complexity of working with perpetrators in an environment where they are not safe and therefore highly restricted in their ability to participate in the normal prison regime.

Consistency and openness

I have found that a consistent and open approach permits men to make further disclosures as work progresses. It is important to reiterate at frequent intervals with clients that their offending was intentional, that they are responsible for their future behaviour and that they can control it. It is then possible to articulate the suspicion that the client has minimised his story whilst acknowledging how difficult it is to tell the truth. A way to help men to address this vital issue is to suggest that one of the barriers to full admission is the need to confront themselves with reality. Having confronted a client with the denial of aspects of his offending, it is then possible to agree to work with what he has disclosed for the time being. It is necessary to remain constantly alert to the opportunity for further disclosure of the offence, and endeavour to create opportunities for this without being unduly persistent.

Challenge and support

Literature on offenders (Garland 1985; Coyle 1991) suggests that imprisonment for many men is counter-productive to change, and social workers need to be aware of this in order to achieve the right balance between challenge and support. Social workers are often seen as 'all things to all people' (Moore and Wood 1992: 148). Men in prison may be isolated both within the prison and in the wider community, especially if their offence has a sexual component. When they see a social worker over an extended period, however unpalatable their offence, a working relationship which requires some element of care for the individual develops. This can be problematic for the client who may feel he will lose support if he divulges the full extent of his offending. It is not helpful for the social worker to be punitive despite the elements of disbelief and confrontation that are important in moving the client forward.

Being able fully to comprehend a situation or circumstance

from another's perspective is both a skill and a personal quality that is an important attribute for a social worker. However, the issue of empathising with a client who has committed a serious crime is clearly fraught with dangers. In order to motivate a response from him, there is a need to create a bridge over which both client and worker can meet. Empathy is possibly one of the most complex issues in the context of working with men. Social workers must develop effective working relationships with their clients, whatever their history, and this necessitates finding ways of engaging which communicate condemnation of the behaviour but not of the individual. Sex offenders for their part find it difficult to empathise, and victim awareness is therefore a key target for intervention.

While support and empathy may be a part of the social work task within prisons, so is the imperative to challenge. Challenging sexism is a routine part of the job. This is more complex within the prison as many sexist beliefs are not untypical of the male population as a whole and therefore likely to be shared by male prison staff and prisoners alike. This could be in terms of role expectations of women as mothers, housewives, carers, or more insidiously as sex objects. For me the most useful way of challenging these views is to present alternatives, asking men to look at what they are saying in terms of the equalness of human beings and encouraging them to look at issues from a woman's position. Essentially the debate must be opened in a non-aggressive manner and discussion invited. A successful debate is more likely without hostility. This is obviously more feasible in situations where there is a continuing relationship rather than in one-off encounters.

The institutionalised attitudes of men towards women in an enclosed male environment are sometimes in conflict with rehabilitative aims which stress the need for men to address aspects of their offending behaviour. Frequently, for example, the Parole Board recommends that a prisoner examines his attitudes and relationships with women. This represents a formal recognition of the problem and yet issues such as the display of sexual images of women within the prison are not tackled in a more general way.[2]

Education

Part of the task of challenging men's perceptions of women is to present an alternative view. Social work in prison offers considerable scope to do this both in terms of intervention strategy and in order to meet the demand for welfare. Women in the outside world are frequently the main support of men in prison. Even when everyone else has given up, there is usually a mother who continues to provide support. In spite of all the other pressures facing women, they struggle to visit, often to be confronted with the outburst of a week's pent-up tension. The mismatch of need at visiting time is frequently vast, and men have little awareness of the realities for their partners or families. Life for many prisoners loses its normal time scale, and the desire for immediate gratification of need becomes intensified. Thus relationships are often subjected to enormous pressure. It is part of the re-education process for social workers to enable prisoners to analyse this process, and put it in the context of gendered power relationships.

Although my male colleagues are aware of these issues, it seems inescapable that the male client perceives me as a greater authority on what it is to be a woman and is perhaps more prepared to hear what I say about the situation for women. A simple but highly illustrative example centres on a discussion between a prisoner and his partner who was telephoning from a maternity hospital where she had just given birth to their child. The man was pressurising the woman to bring the baby into the prison without delay and seemed to be meeting some resistance. He asked me to speak to his partner on the telephone. She quickly conveyed to me her physical discomfort following a difficult delivery, which I then explained to her partner. He was prepared to listen to a detailed description of the effects of childbirth and modified his approach to his partner accordingly. Clearly, an alternative approach in this case might have been to encourage the female partner to be more assertive, but tackling the man's perceptions seems to have worked equally well.

Power and control

Control is a significant feature of abusive behaviour, and, from my discussions with male colleagues and students, is clearly an issue that presents difficulties for both male and female workers. Sex offenders are adept at finding weaknesses in whoever they are trying to control or manipulate. The social worker has to recognise personal weaknesses and strive to reinforce these areas if she is to maintain control of an interview.

Lloyd Sinclair, addressing the 1991 ROTA Conference,[3] stressed the need for workers to present themselves as extremely confident when working with sex offenders. Experience is obviously an asset in this; however, it is also about workers mentally reinforcing themselves before they start. It is vital to plan the interview, set objectives for the session, anticipate the difficult areas, clarify possible strategies, and think about the traps. My experience is that time for reflection before the interview improves self-confidence and allows the worker to take control of the interview. This element is so vital and yet easy to overlook in the pressure of a busy working day. Lack of preparation leads to loss of control, and this may take the work backwards rather than forwards. There are, however, useful strategies for regaining control, sometimes lost as a result of losing concentration. One is to change the immediate focus of the discussion by asking a question about a different, although related, topic. Another is to ask for considerable detail about what the client is relating, thus making him respond to you rather than maintain his control of the interview.

I believe that there may at times be a dichotomy between the social worker's requirement to assist an offender in addressing his offending behaviour and the need perceived by many prisoners and prison staff for help and counselling with the relationship problems which are almost synonymous with imprisonment. However, if offending is viewed as part of the total situation in which a person exists, and especially if the victim of the offence is a woman, there can be a strong connection between offending behaviour and relationship problems. This is particularly significant in the area of control. In entering prison a man loses control of most aspects of his life. Very often this leads him to strive even harder to maintain control over his home life. This can involve making excessive demands on his family to involve him in their decision-making. Although this may be acceptable to some women, many women discover that they can manage households, budgeting and the children equally well without their partner. This inevitably shifts the power dynamics in their relationship, creating huge problems for a man who has already lost control of his life. He must learn therefore that he does not have to dominate to have a successful relationship, and that there is merit in allowing his partner to grow into a whole person. This challenge to the machismo (which is frequently linked to recidivist behaviour) can provide a valuable adjunct to other interventions.

One of the prerequisites to controlling inappropriate behaviour is to acknowledge that behaviour in full, and much of the purpose of intervention is directed towards breaking down denial and minimisation. Thus I return repeatedly to discussion of the offence, encouraging the man to offer more detail. I have found this approach successful in reducing denial of abusing behaviour and have had significant revelations months after initiating contact. I expect this process to take time in view of the complex and secret nature of sexual behaviour. Although we have not got all the time in the world to effect some change, it does seem highly improbable that behaviours that have taken years to establish are going to yield to a few challenging encounters with a social worker. Nevertheless, I have found that a strategy of persistence, consistency and support over time has enabled men with entrenched patterns of thinking to move forward particularly in the areas of cognitive distortions, denial and victim awareness. Undoubtedly, intensive programmes based on cognitive behavioural techniques can have a significant impact over short periods (Marshall and Barbaree 1990), but even intensive programmes in ideal conditions such as at the Gracewell Clinic lasted for a year and staff would have preferred longer (Renvoize 1993).

Gender awareness

An awareness of gender and traditional male/female roles adds to the complexity of intervention strategies for women working with male clients. It provides a powerful tool in developing empathy and in challenging distorted thinking. It is not the male client alone who may have difficulty in comprehending the reality of situations from the victim's perspective. Prison staff may also experience this. At a training exercise for prison and social work staff, a woman survivor of a sexual attack related in graphic detail how she was beaten over the head with the poker and then forced to have oral sex.[4] The response from my male colleagues was dramatic. They were visibly emotionally shattered, and evidently altered in their attitudes during the remainder of the course. From appearing to pay lip-service to the need to develop ways to help men address their inappropriate and violent behaviour to women and children they became vehement protagonists. It is this ability for women to express to men the impact of their behaviour on women that is one of the key features of being a woman doing this work. This can be particularly helpful if a cognitive behavioural approach is used when the aim is to challenge the thinking patterns that create the cognitive distortions which condone the abusive behaviour. Men are undoubtedly very successful in this type of work, but I believe that women are advantaged by nature of their gender. Women's experience of early conditioning generates an awareness of the power imbalance in the relationships between men and women. A woman's understanding of the power imbalance in tackling victim awareness with male perpetrators can also be transferred to child victims. Thus power and control are a valuable focus for women working with men.

Language and touch

A hurdle which must be overcome in work with sex offenders is how to discuss explicit sexual matters. However open we are ourselves about sex, our culture tends to imbue such discourse with overtones of intimacy or smut rather than fact or biology. This can provide a difficult barrier for both worker and client. Nevertheless, in order to engage the client in direct work about his offence, we must develop the ability to discuss sex in as straightforward a manner as if it were nothing more than a shopping transaction.

Familiarity undoubtedly reduces the impact of talking about sex. But it is important to acknowledge the impact of the worker's own sexual conditioning which might at times lead to a flicker of sexual response to the language of explicit sexual discussion, unrelated to the context of the interview. Working with sex offenders challenges workers to reassess their own sexuality, and we must find ways of being comfortable with this. In analysing personal issues in relation to sex, the recognition that violent and bizarre sexual behaviour exists on the extreme end of the same continuum as conventional sexual behaviour can be a source of great confusion.

Perhaps surprisingly, this realisation is itself an important step in enabling the worker to acknowledge the 'humanness' of the sex offender. Without either condoning or minimising the offender's behaviour the worker needs to demonstrate acceptance of him as a human being with hope for the future.

I am struck by the ways in which my approach to the issue of explicit sexual discussion with men mirrors the 'grooming' process which the sex offender utilises with his young victims. Difficult areas are introduced slowly, perhaps only touching the issue fleetingly the first time, to return and take it further subsequently. In this way the topic becomes more comfortable, and both the worker and the client are more confident about the discussion. This is not suggested as the only way to work, but is offered as an effective means to enabling some men to vocalise the sexual aspects of their behaviour simply and directly.

Working with men in this environment has also made me conscious of the issues around physical touch. There are many ways of helping people, men or women, to deal with grief and the worker can find touch an appropriate means of supportive, non-verbal communication. In an environment where men are largely deprived of nurturing, physical contact, their senses are heightened. It is therefore helpful to be particularly careful to avoid providing any sensory stimulation either by touch, smell or dress. Whilst this means that the environment is essentially controlling the presentation of self, this is in effect a dual-edged response; both a sensitivity to male imprisonment and a personal protection.

Potential for violence

The widespread expectation is that working in a prison places a social worker in a vulnerable position with regard to violence. However, although an awareness that violence is a possibility remains on the daily agenda, it has not been my general experience during the last four years at Edinburgh. Here an apparently well-established, stable situation exists within the prison as a whole. That is not to say that there is no violence among the prisoners, but that as a social worker, your situation is generally well-controlled, and you are not in the highly vulnerable situation experienced by many social workers doing a home visit. It is important to recognise this because it may influence your perception of an individual's dangerousness and provide you with the potential for cognitive distortion. People who commit horrendous offences look just like anyone else, and, their offending behaviour aside, most often communicate and relate just like anyone else. Thus for the prison-based social worker, prisoners can present a very unreal persona, certainly away from the hall situation.

Nevertheless, prisoners can and do at times communicate their violence without directing it at the social worker. For example, men without histories of violent behaviour will talk about violent retributive acts they plan to make. There is aggression in their tone of voice, facial expression and body language. The social worker's task is to recognise what is reality and what is fantasy, and to challenge them with this. Men can frequently demonstrate a controlled violence about situations that cause frustration or anger. Allowing space for this explosion of tension can have a therapeutic element as well as providing issues to work with. In general, a low-key, non-confrontational approach is the most effective response when faced with an angry man. It can also be helpful with some men to discuss the fact that their manner frightens people and look at alternative strategies for getting what they want, or accepting what they cannot have. This itself is a form of assertiveness training.

Co-working

Limited resources and a burgeoning number of imprisoned sex offenders inhibit the development of co-working. I have only been able to work with a colleague on one occasion. This was a positive experience for both the client and the workers involved, and moved the client forward more quickly than subsequent work with individuals. Notwithstanding my male colleague's experience and ability, the paired interview overcame very effectively the issue of control, releasing the workers from a familiar difficulty. Interviewing in a small group like this also provided a less intimate situation in which to discuss sexual matters.

PERSONAL ISSUES IN DIRECT WORK WITH MEN

Does a diet full of substantially disturbing crime, mostly against women, have an effect on the female worker? Undoubtedly my work has had a considerable effect on me and at times has made me question my motivation and strength to continue. During my first months in the prison I was plagued by mental images of the more significant crimes that I heard about, made all the more real by contact with the perpetrator. However, two conclusions have emerged for me.

First, despite considerable initial trauma I have kept going without any apparently negative long-term effects on me as a person outside my work. The sensitivity that work with sex offenders requires seems to heighten personal sensitivity, making the work both painful and challenging. Nevertheless, the struggle of working with this can itself be a helpful ingredient in improving social work skills, through maintaining the balance between challenge and support.

Second, work with the perpetrators of crime (mainly men) is an essential element of protecting the women and children who are most frequently the victims of sexual assaults. As my knowledge has increased, so has my confidence that the skills required to change men *can* be developed, providing there is both commitment and opportunity.

There are two issues which remain unresolved as yet for me, and need exploration. Fantasy is a significant ingredient in the sexual offender's cycle of abuse. Fantasy is also a normal human occupation. As a woman working in a predominantly male environment it is necessary to acknowledge, at least intellectually, the fact that you may be the object of male fantasy. This possibility is not something normally dwelt on in a significant way except to identify the issue and intellectualise it. The reality of having such a situation confirmed is an unpleasant experience and challenges both your capacity to deal with the issue appropriately and your ability to cope with the intrusion into your personal space. For a woman working through such issues to be faced with only male supervision can be both inhibiting and extremely limited in terms of support.

It is also important to consider the direct impact of hearing about serious, particularly sexual, crimes. There is feeling of contamination in this, which creates some of the initial personal trauma in working with sex offenders. In my early experiences of hearing the detail of violent crime I experienced something similar to a 'flash-back' at inappropriate moments outside my work. For a while this undoubtedly had an effect on my usual responses as a woman. I have discussed this with male colleagues who did not seem to have had similar experiences. As the victim of many of the sexual crimes is female, it is perhaps not possible for a man to put himself in the place of the victim.

And yet this is not the whole picture. I am also conscious of positive personal by-products of my work with men in prison. Openness, confidence and personal insight are attributes that develop as a result of meeting the challenge of this work. I have found this development of self only helpful in the task of being human.

FINAL THOUGHTS

It is clear from what I have said already that the dynamics of working with male prisoners are inextricably linked with the male ethos in the prison as a whole. It becomes a complex task, therefore, to separate the gender issues of the workplace from clients' gender issues or indeed from the structural issues of working within a large, male-dominated organisation. I met my personal 'Waterloo' at an early stage in my prison career. I was interviewing a prisoner in the interview room on the hall and had been interrupted several times in the space of a few minutes by a prison officer. When the same officer came in a further time to find out when I would be finished as the doctor (male) wanted the room, I responded fairly sharply by saying 'When I am ready!' After the interview the officer returned to the room, backed me against the wall and bawled me out for undermining his authority in front of a prisoner. I suspect that he would neither have harassed me nor verbally attacked me had I been a man, and that it was my response in front of the prisoner as a woman that particularly incensed him. This story had a positive ending in that, having collected my wits and with the support of my male manager, I was able to confront the officer publicly, which did much to increase my credibility. These power challenges are an everyday occurrence although thankfully seldom so extreme.

Feminist women working in a male prison can feel overwhelmed at the size of the task in attempting to change men's behaviour. Promoting feminist ideas as a direct tool of social work intervention with men does need to be clearly on the agenda. In the process of writing this chapter I have become more aware of my position in relation to feminism and conscious that I do not acknowledge this in any significant way with colleagues. I am also aware that the challenge of analysing my practice has had a developmental effect, so that I am no longer writing from the same position as when I started. Although this inevitably creates some problems, it nevertheless demonstrates the value of close examination of practice. Work with sex offenders has to be clearly focused, with considerable direction and planning. The challenge of meeting this demand undoubtedly has value for all other social work intervention (Lupton and Gillespie 1994).

The task of challenging men to view the world from a pro-feminist perspective seems a daunting, even unrealisable, goal. Working in isolation with relatively few prisoners or male officers seems rather like trying to hold the sea back. Perhaps the best hope may lie in the cascade effect – that your impact on some men will have a subsidiary effect on others. In this way, the process of changing men's attitudes and behaviour towards women will continue.

NOTES

1 Central government introduced 100 per cent funding for social work services with offenders in Scotland in April 1991. The National Objectives and Standards for Social Work in the Criminal Justice System prepared by the Social Work Services Group were published in the same year to coincide with this and to provide detailed guidance for practice.
2 Certain institutions which are seeking to work directly with sexual offenders demand an acceptance of pornography-free living situations.
3 Regional Offender Treatment Association which in 1991, following rapid development, became a national association for the development of work with sex offenders known as NOTA. The aim is to provide a forum for learning, and development for those working in the field of sexual offending. Lloyd Sinclair, Attic Correctional Services, Wisconsin, social worker, psychotherapist and sex therapist, was a key speaker at the ROTA Conference, 1991, at Liverpool University.
4 I am very appreciative of the contribution made by 'Judy' to widen both public and ministerial awareness of the plight of victims of sexual attacks, and I am grateful for her permission to include her story.

Chapter 3

Working with the CHANGE men's programme

Monica Wilson

Since September 1989, I have worked as joint co-ordinator of the CHANGE project,[1] a pro-feminist organisation which runs a criminal justice-based re-education programme for male perpetrators of domestic violence. My tasks as joint co-ordinator involve me in a substantial amount of direct contact with violent men, including compiling court reports assessing men's suitability for the programme and co-facilitating the programme's group-work sessions. This chapter will briefly describe the origins and development of the CHANGE men's programme. This will be followed by a discussion of some of the issues involved for me, as a feminist, working with men. This is a personal and experiential account, and whilst it probably raises more questions than it answers about the role of women working in men's programmes, it nevertheless charts some of the very real dilemmas which I have struggled with in the course of my involvement with CHANGE.

UNDERSTANDING DOMESTIC VIOLENCE

Despite over two decades of research, countless academic books and scholarly papers, we did not have to look very far for an understanding of why men are violent to the women with whom they live. Most of us grew up with an understanding that women should know their place and if they did not, men would show them. We learned from an early age that the freedom boys enjoyed was denied to us. We were told that the world was a dangerous place for girls and women and that we would need a man to protect us from those dangers. And, although we understood that men should not hit women, if a husband hit his wife we were led to believe she had deserved it.

The feminist understanding of domestic violence that women have struggled to elucidate comes from the pain and anguish of personal experience. Since the early 1970s women activists and their allies have campaigned for the recognition of the nature, extent and impact of the problem of domestic violence on women's lives and have worked to provide safety and support for the victims of men's violence. This has involved the provision of refuges for women and their children, challenging institutional and community tolerance of men's violence to women and campaigning for social change and legal reform (Schechter 1982; Dobash and Dobash 1992).

However, until recently, men have been shielded from the full focus of attention on their behaviour because of the way in which theories of the causes of domestic violence have developed. Following the rediscovery of the problem in the early 1970s, initial theories developed from research which concentrated on the pathology or deviance of individual victims and perpetrators (Schultz 1960; Faulk 1973; Gayford 1975). Later, as the flaws and inadequacies of these explanation were highlighted (Dobash and Dobash 1979), the focus was broadened to include wider social, structural and cultural factors (Goode 1971; Gelles 1972; Steinmetz and Straus 1974). As the first approach blamed individual victims, then perpetrators, so the next perspective blamed society (Smith 1989). Neither approach offered a satisfactory explanation for men's violence to women. Extending the analysis further, feminist researchers included the concept of patriarchy and the imbalance of power in male–female relationships as being central to explaining domestic violence (Dobash and Dobash 1979; Adams 1988; Bograd 1988; Dobash and Dobash 1992).

Theories which explain domestic violence in terms of the psychopathologies of either the men or women have received lasting attention in the United States. Some academics and activists describe the United States as a 'therapeutic society' (Dobash and Dobash 1992: 216) which sees therapy as the solution to almost all social, economic and political problems. The political attractiveness of explanations which focus on treating 'sick' individuals rather than addressing the need for wider social or institutional change have contributed to the growth of therapeutic discourses which have transformed perceptions of domestic violence.

Similarly, the 'discovery' by American researchers (Steinmetz 1978) that men could be the victims of spouse abuse just as much as women, implied that the problem was an evenly balanced one and that solutions lay in therapeutic interventions on an interpersonal or familial level. In the United States there has been fierce debate between family violence researchers and pro-feminist researchers about their different approaches to the problem, a debate which continues unabated (Saunders 1988; Dobash and Dobash 1992; Bart and Moran 1993). Although the pro-feminist perspective is influential, it remains a minority view among the other explanations which compete to inform intervention.

In the United Kingdom the feminist perspective has been a dominant influence informing work with abused women and campaigning by activists. The 'solution' to the problem from this perspective lies in challenging the historical legacy of patriarchal idealogy which fosters the acceptance of gender as 'natural' or 'God-given' rather than socially constructed (Dobash and Dobash 1979; Scully 1990). By placing domestic violence in its historical, cultural and situational contexts, the pro-feminist perspective offers a broad theory of the problem which can account for the question 'why do men use physical force against their wives' (Bograd 1988: 21). Put simply, men abuse their partners because they have been permitted, even encouraged, to do so for centuries. Many continue to believe they still have the right to use physical chastisement to dominate and control their partners.

SO WHY WORK WITH MEN?

At the time that CHANGE was being developed, there was a growing debate in the United Kingdom about the principle of working with men. Some feminists viewed the development of this work with alarm. There are many persuasive arguments for *not* working with men. For example, issues of scarce resources, the refocusing of the political agenda, the possibility of increased danger to women and giving women false hope (Hart 1988; Hague and Malos 1993) are all pertinent here.

Once men's work started being resourced, it was feared, work with women and children survivors of their crimes would suffer. Politicians would be able to say that this was the avenue for reform that was now being pursued and that women would no longer need refuge and support as men would stop being violent. Also, given the attraction of these new ideas, work with men was likely to invite far more media attention than the continuing struggle to keep work with women and children on the public agenda.

Others have argued that the work is far too dangerous and could seriously harm women, and that even if a man's physical violence stops as a result of attending a programme, he may learn better 'terroristic tactics' (Hart 1988: 67). In addition, by offering a man an avenue whereby he must state his intention to reform, his partner may be robbed of her moment of escape. Most women have heard men say all too often that they did not mean it and that it will not happen again; that they will change. Frequently women will have refrained from calling the police or seeking other help because they want to believe that their partner could change.

Women have to overcome many obstacles when invoking the law over domestic violence. They might be asked if they want the man to be charged, which makes many women think it is their responsibility for charges being laid. They will have to maintain their evidence often over a long period of time and not succumb to pressure for charges to be dropped. They may have to face the stigma of publicity. The moment where a man's responsibility for his violence has been announced publicly by a conviction in a court of law is a crucial time in a woman's life. At such a time she may find the strength to decide that she must get away from him. At this time too she may well have made contact with services that can help her make that transition. By offering her partner a place on a men's programme, that process may be temporarily halted; she may feel that perhaps this time he *will* change and she may postpone the decision to leave. Arguably therefore, we should not even contemplate working with men. They should be properly punished, and we should concentrate on campaigning for change and the empowerment of women through the provision of access to education, jobs and decent childcare services.

Powerful though these arguments may be, and appealing as they are to the sense of indignation over women's subjugation, other feminists, myself included, believe that we do need to work with men (Pence and Shepard 1988). Focusing on campaigns and changing women and women's circumstances alone will not be sufficient to end men's violence, because such strategies by themselves will not relieve men of their power. Men's power has remained largely untouched and unaltered by feminism. Stopping men's violence means altering the balance of power between men and women on individual, institutional and societal levels. We need to challenge violent men, and traditional social and institutional tolerance of their violence. We need to challenge the *status quo* and men's understanding of their place in the world. We need men to question and change the ways in which they grow up to believe that they have certain rights over women which they can enforce.

The most persuasive argument for working with men is that many abused women *want* this work to take place. Although refuge and support is crucial for women who want to leave a violent partner, not all women want to make that break. Many will stay, hoping the violence will stop. They are prepared to give men a chance to change. Intervention programmes for violent men have a part to play in bringing about this change and can complement the work being undertaken by those providing support services for women and children. Programmes must be aware of the potential danger to women; they must take serious account of this through the provision of support services and responsible working practices.

DEVELOPING THE CHANGE PROJECT

By the mid-1980s, it had become clear in the United Kingdom that, among other moves towards more active intervention with offenders, there was interest from the voluntary and statutory agencies in looking at ways of addressing men's violence to women. In North America work with men had been in existence for a decade or more, much of it therapeutic in approach (Eisikovits and Edleson 1989). There were fears among activists in the United Kingdom that, following the maxim that what happens in the United States yesterday happens here tomorrow, such programmes might be imported by the voluntary or statutory agencies and established here.

A small number of pro-feminist projects in North America were, however, operating men's programmes as part of a co-ordinated community response to domestic violence (Edleson *et al.* 1985; Pence and Shepard 1988; Sinclair 1989). These projects placed men's programmes within a wider context so that work with men was seen to serve a greater purpose than changing the individual; it was part of a process of enhancing community responses to men's violence to women and influencing institutional responses. While the research evidence of the effectiveness of this form of intervention was in its early days (Pirog-Good and Stets-Kealy 1985; Edleson and Syers 1989), this was the type of model that activists thought might offer the best approach to work with men in the United Kingdom. The CHANGE project in Scotland was intended to pilot such work and had the support of Scottish Women's Aid, albeit with many of the aforementioned reservations.

SETTING THE CONTEXT

The CHANGE men's programme begins from the premise that men's violence to women partners is behaviour which they have learned in the context of our patriarchal culture, their socialisation as men and their personal experiences. It is neither natural nor inevitable, but cultural in origin. As learned behaviour it is underpinned by the attitudes and beliefs inherent in patriarchy. At its simplest it can be summarised as the belief that women are inferior and subservient to men, particularly in the context of personal relationships, and that men have certain rights over women. Those rights can be asserted or enforced through a range of coercive behaviour culminating in the use of physical force. The work undertaken with men proposes that men must change their attitudes, beliefs and associated behaviours if they are to live non-violently with women partners.

Following the co-ordinated community approach of the North American models which have informed our practice, the CHANGE men's programme was designed to operate within the criminal justice system. Men are referred to the programme as a condition of a probation order, following the preparation of court reports, including a report from CHANGE which assesses their suitability for the programme.[2] Social workers, in their capacity as probation officers, supervise the orders.

Locating the work within the justice system is intended to impact not just on violent men, but also on the institutions which dispense justice. The criminal nature of men's violence to their partners has often been underplayed in the past by the police, prosecutors and sentencers (Wasoff 1982; Faragher 1985; Johnson 1985b; Pahl 1985). The message given by the criminal justice system to women, men and the community is a vital part of the response to male violence, and may either serve to reinforce the idea that wife abuse is a private matter or that violence against any member of the community is an offence deserving an effective response from the justice system in co-ordination with other agencies of the state and the community (Morran and Wilson 1994).

The most obvious response, and one that many feminist activists support, is to call for the justice system to use custodial sentences for crimes of violence to women (Edwards 1989). This, it is argued, would spell out very clearly that violence to women was being treated seriously and severely. At the same time, however, we know that prison does little or nothing to challenge offending behaviour and effect personal change (Home Office 1990). Although it may offer some respite from the physical abuse, and provide some space during which women can look at their options, there is growing awareness among probation officers and social workers that while in prison men are often able to exert considerable pressure on women through the use of family networks and visits. In addition, many abused women do not want their partner to go to prison, and the fear that this could happen may deter some women from reporting the violence in the first place (Hague and Malos 1993).

CHANGE supports the position that, in some cases, the prison option may be appropriate for emphasising the seriousness of violence to women. However, experience demonstrates that the majority of such offenders are given non-custodial disposals and, in these cases CHANGE offers a new sentencing option. By making attendance at the men's programme contingent upon charge, prosecution and conviction, and carrying the sanction of a probation condition, the criminal nature of domestic violence is emphasised and this communicates a very important message to the community.

FEATURES OF THE CHANGE MEN'S PROGRAMME

At the time when we were working to develop the programme, research evidence concerning the effectiveness of programmes was patchy but indicated that short, educationally focused, structured programmes appeared to be most effective in reducing men's violent and abusive behaviour to their partners (Pirog-Good and Stets-Kealy 1985; Eisikovits and Edleson 1989; Edleson and Tolman 1992). The CHANGE men's programme has an educational-style curriculum and is highly structured. It operates using a modular approach, and men are required to attend sixteen to twenty-two sessions in order to complete the programme.

The programme has four main goals:

1 To increase men's awareness that their violence and abuse is intentional and not mysterious behaviour, and that they alone are responsible for their violent behaviour and for changing it.
2 To challenge the attitudes and beliefs that underlie that behaviour.
3 To develop skills to live in a non-abusive partnership with women.
4 To monitor individual men's progress through record-keeping and reports to social workers, partners and courts.

Men sign a contract called the Agreement to Participate which clearly outlines the rules and requirements of the programme. Breaking or failing to comply with any of them constitutes grounds for a breach of the probation order. When this occurs, the CHANGE coordinators report the transgression to the supervising social worker who will formally instigate breach procedures. The final sanction remains with the courts.

CONTACT WITH WOMEN PARTNERS

The CHANGE policy in relation to the women partners of the men on the programme is based on two premises: first, that women's safety *must* be the prime consideration when deciding men's suitability for the programme; and second, that once on the programme, women are entitled to information both about the nature and content of the work and their partner's progress. We also recognise that women have needs of their own. CHANGE has insufficient resources to provide a service to women, so in practice this has resulted in trying to work with other agencies in a flexible and collaborative way to adjust to women's changing needs and circumstances. For example, currently CHANGE, social work, Women's Aid, and the police are working together to provide a support group for women partners. This also operates as a springboard for them to find out about other local resources.

DILEMMAS AND RESPONSES

In this section I will concentrate on my work in the men's programme, exploring some of the dilemmas I have struggled with as a feminist working with men. Such issues include joint facilitation, confronting and challenging men, possible pitfalls encountered in this work and the effects of hearing misogynous talk. I will then discuss the impact the work has had on me, and finally I want to look at what I believe are the positive and constructive aspects of this work.

Women as joint facilitators

The issue of joint facilitation of men's programmes has been debated for a number of years, particularly in North America. One school of thought argues that, since this is a problem for which men are responsible, men must take sole responsibility for doing the work to change themselves. Involving women in the programmes can communicate the message that women are taking some of that responsibility. A counter-argument questions whether women can trust men to do this work themselves. Women's involvement is seen as important to 'police' the agenda and ensure that programmes do not become male bonding groups with workers being drawn into collusion with men's excuses for violence (Hart 1988).

I believe that the involvement of women in this work is important for two main reasons. The first is centred on keeping women's perspective and experience of the world, and of men, on the agenda at group sessions. Another, more importantly, has to do with confronting men with the impact their behaviour has on their partners, both in terms of physical pain and injury, and in terms of emotional pain and psychological damage.

I would also argue that men and women bring different but equally valuable perspectives into the group. They can demonstrate and model an equal relationship, and can show methods of discussing disagreements which do not use abuse. However, it should not be supposed that this is an easy task to accomplish, nor that men will necessarily relate what they see modelled as relevant to their lives. Issues of social class, background and the dichotomy of personal and professional roles all intervene.

There are some ways in which it is relatively easy to model an equal relationship with my male colleague. We can make clear statements that we are co-workers, neither of us in charge of the other. We alternate certain housekeeping tasks such as answering administrative questions, leading the group introduction and closing exercises and handing out bus fares to those who qualify for them. But there are some aspects of the curriculum which I have come to recognise are less easy to handle in an even-handed way, particularly when the sessions involve confronting and challenging men's excuses and justifications for their violence and talking about the beliefs which underpin these.

Confronting and challenging men

Challenging men begins in the early stages of the programme when they are asked to look at the range of explanations which they may have used over time to justify their violent and abusive behaviours to their partners. Mostly these explanations are couched in language which justifies or excuses their behaviour. Words like 'provocation', 'drink' or 'loss of control' are commonplace. These are then re-examined and the ways in which men use denial, blame and minimisation as techniques for shifting responsibility and reducing feelings of guilt are explored in depth. Using case-study examples, men can usually identify how other men use denial, blame and minimisation, but find it much more difficult to accept that their own 'reasons' are in fact excuses. Many are keen to portray themselves as 'victims' of their partner's irrational behaviour or disobedience. If only *she* would just 'do what she's told', 'shut up when I tell her', 'know when to stop', 'listen to me', then none of this would have happened. They will sometimes endorse one another's statements. It is crucial that they are constantly told that it is not their partner's behaviour that is at issue, but their behaviour; they are the one with the criminal conviction; and their explanations are the rationalisations which are not acceptable.

Further work on men's attitudes and beliefs, about themselves as men and about women, follows. My male colleague can challenge the group and invoke his own experience as a man growing up in the same culture as them and the shared experience of men's attitudes to women. This makes it harder for the men to dismiss his reasoning as nonsense or as irrelevant to them, although many will want to argue and debate with him.

It is my experience that challenges about attitudes and behaviour have more validity for some men when they come from another man. When a challenge does come from me I have been aware that at times it is not taken as seriously as when it comes from my male colleague, or at least not until he has endorsed it. The dismissal of my challenge can take the form of verbal responses such as me being 'just' another woman who 'doesn't understand'; or taunts that I am a 'women's libber'. These can be confronted to some extent by my colleague's endorsing what I have said or repeating my question. More diffi-cult to counter are the subtle signals of body language; the shifting in the chair (especially a man sliding down the chair and thrusting his crotch at you), the blank or mocking facial expression, gazes lifted to the ceiling, glances exchanged among them, exasperated sighs.

The realisation that some men can use the strategy of dismiss-ing *my* views as irrelevant or amusing is very undermining and has occasionally had the effect of instantly disempowering me in the group. Such experiences are not constant and usually occur during the early stages of the programme when some men are still resistant to being in the group. As I have become more experienced in the work this still occurs but has become less of a problem for me. Not because men no longer try to dismiss my views, or to undermine me in other ways, but because I am more alert to their likely responses, and so I am less thrown by them. Sometimes I can even circumvent them by telling them in advance how I expect them to react. The key to coping here, as in so many aspects of this work, is preparation.

Being the woman in the group, I am on the other hand, able to talk about women's viewpoints and experience; something a man could not do as convincingly. I am also better placed to confront men with the impact their behaviour has had on their partner and in this I can invoke my experience. My colleague sometimes needs to seek *my* endorsement when he refers to women's experience.

The men I have worked with, and perhaps men in general, seem to have little idea of how women experience the world and are minimally motivated to want to understand women's viewpoint. Women, conversely, grow up in a society in which men's view of the world predominates (Spender 1980). We do an exercise in the group where men are asked to list, first, the qualities and skills which boys are traditionally taught to see as important as they become men and, second, the qualities and skills which girls are taught to see as important for women. We then look at the sanctions placed on men and women to conform to their respective roles. The exercise serves two purposes: to look at how men are desensitised by the process of socialisation and how they are taught to perceive women as subservient; and to explore the ways in which women's freedoms are limited in the process of their socialisation. Once the men in the group perceive the intent of the exercise, some of them will argue heatedly that women differ from men only when it comes to having children. Far from being treated as inferior, women, as some of them see it, are in a privileged position and 'have it all their own way'. At times like this, a woman can try to provide a (pro-)feminist lens for the men, offering her view about how women experience the world. I have found that, in time, the hostility of some men towards hearing this can be diminished as men begin to realise that the world cannot continue to revolve around them and that some consideration of the needs and views of their partners can, potentially, positively affect their own lives. In my experience some members of the group are more receptive to these ideas and will argue with the other men; occasionally group pressure shifts the perspectives of the more intransigent ones.

Confronting men with the impact their violence and abuse has had on their partners, on children and other family members is something I believe a woman is better placed to do than a man. I can talk with validity about women's physical hurt and injuries, and about emotional pain and fear. Men are taught not to identify with and even actively to suppress such emotions (Rubin 1983). Moreover, by citing my own experience and relating it to how I think I would feel if I was their partner, I can push them and even play on their developing feelings of guilt in a way which might bring more vocal resentment if it came from a man.

It is a constant source of surprise to me how little men understand the damage they do to those they profess to love. The remorse that we often hear from them has usually more to do with the pain they are feeling for themselves and resentment for their criminal conviction. Empathy for their partner and remorse for what they have done to her is relatively rare. What remorse there may be is often coupled with sharing out blame with her for having got them into this trouble.

Some possible pitfalls

When you know what a man has done to his partner there is the temptation sometimes to punish him. You may deceive yourself into thinking that what you are doing is challenging him. We need to learn to recognise the difference between challenging a man in a supportive and constructive way and being so confrontational that he feels humiliated and threatened by you. My concern is not so much that the man may feel bad and emotionally upset; sometimes that is an important part of the process of his becoming more aware of how he behaves. Rather, I am concerned that on leaving the group he will resent having been humiliated (and sometimes by a woman), and either reject the programme message, or, much more seriously, take it out on his partner. It is important that each session ends in such a way that emotions raised have been properly processed and men leave in a positive frame of mind.

Conversely, there is the pitfall of trying to be liked by the men. Partly I think this has to do with my upbringing as a woman; I was taught to be 'nice' to others, and to men in particular (Baker Miller 1978). While I am aware of this possibility, it is sometimes difficult to resist. There is another dimension, however. Many of the men I work with *are* likeable; indeed, this can often be one of their partner's complaints: 'He's so charming when we're out together that people don't believe he hits me.' I have to remind myself constantly why I am in the same room as these men and what my task is. As for the more recalcitrant men, there is the danger of trying to 'charm' them into opening up more.

While there needs to be some rapport and cooperation between workers and men for learning to take place, it is important to be alert to the danger of men feeling that you are 'on their side', and that you 'understand'. If you present as sympathetic and willing to listen it can all too easily drift into collusion.

As well as being alert to the danger of trying to be liked, I am also aware now that at the start of this work I willed the men to 'see the light' and I worked hard for them. I was so committed to making the programme work. At the end of each two-and-a-half-hour session I was exhausted but felt I had worked well. I have since become more aware of the need to step back from too intense an involvement with the group. It is up to the men to do the work; not me.

Being the woman worker means that occasionally I have become caught up in individual women's crises after they have contacted me for advice and assistance. Information about a man's violent or abusive behaviour may be revealed to me in confidence. Despite many years of experience, I have not yet, and hopefully never will, become inured to hearing women relate the horror of their abuse by men. Sometimes this has had a devastating effect on my ability to do my main task which is to work with the man. I no longer trust his motivation to change, nor that of the others in the group. I question the whole point of working with men. While this can be personally undermining, it is not necessarily a bad thing. It is important that workers on men's programmes are constantly reminded of the reality for abused women. The work has to be accountable to women, and they should have opportunities to inform workers of continuing abuse so that appropriate action can be taken. It is essential that we question what we are doing and do not become complacent.

Hearing misogyny

Most of the men I have worked with profess to love and respect their partners and some profess to treat them as equals. They will counter any suggestion that they do not with assertions that they do the hoovering or the cooking. But in reality, their opinion of women is woefully low. One of the exercises men do in the early stages of the programme requires them to list two things they most like and two they most dislike about being a man. While this is seen by most as an extremely difficult exercise to address ('I've just never thought about things this way'), after some discussion, by far the majority state the first thing they most like about being a man is not being a woman.[3] Perhaps this is hardly surprising given that most feminine characteristics are exactly those which boys are taught to reject. When asked to qualify their answer most find it difficult with the exception of the horror of having babies.

Hearing men's misogyny is made more difficult by the fact that they are not aware of it and deeply resent the suggestion that they are women-haters. But it is communicated most clearly through their use of language. Men have to be reminded continually that their partner has a name; they will refer to her as 'her' or 'the wife'. They will refer to other women in terms which, while undoubtedly colloquial, are also derogatory; 'bint' or 'doll' being but two. When we do exercises which break down individual men's violent attacks on their partners, and look at the man's intent and its relationship to his beliefs and expectations of his partner, the language used is also revealing. Usually it involves both giving orders and delivering deeply degrading sexual insults.

In the group setting, the men are careful to 'show' respect to me as a woman and moderate their language to some extent, but their guard can drop during cigarette breaks when sexist references might be made during talk about pubs, TV programmes or work. Whether to ignore this, or try to make use of it in the group is an unresolved issue. We are not the 'thought police', and we know that this is what they hear all the time away from the group. We can only hope that growing awareness will help them question it in time. Generally we leave men on their own at breaks.

The impact on my life

Inevitably, doing this work has had a tremendous impact on my life, much of it deeply personal. Space does not permit an exhaustive account, and some of it may not even be apparent to me, so I shall summarise what I see as the main features.

One of the hardest consequences for me has been the criticism that, as a woman and a feminist, I am betraying my sisters by 'helping' these despicable violent men. The criticism that by working with men as a feminist I am betraying the cause may not be a very sophisticated one but it does speak to the deepest of gut-felt emotions. I understand where it comes from and should have been prepared for it. I know from personal and professional experience the damage violent men have inflicted and continue to inflict on women. Women's legitimate anger is also my anger. My considered response is that it is indeed *because* I am a feminist that I want to do this work. It would be easier not to. It would not require much courage to stay on the moral high ground of indignation about what men have done, and there is plenty of sisterly support for those who do so. It demands much more to take the challenge to the 'opposition', to men who are the known abusers of women. For too long men have not been held accountable for their behaviour towards women. Domestic violence should not be treated as a 'women's issue', although it is, and has been an issue *for* women for centuries.

For me, working for CHANGE is an opportunity to be in the vanguard of a new way of taking men to task for their violence. It offers a chance to confront and challenge both them, and the institutions and ideology which have permitted, even encouraged, their violence. At the same time it is an optimistic development. Perhaps men *can* change. It is worth attempting. Not all men are violent; many abhor violence. Some are allies in the feminist cause (Hearn 1987; Brod 1987; Connell 1987; Morgan 1992). I am not, however, working to 'help' violent men, but to help abused women. I do this work because I want men to stop their violence to women, and because I want men to be held responsible for their behaviour towards their partners and for stopping it. But as a consequence I am conscious of feeling isolated from some feminists, and I am saddened by that.

There is no doubt too that the work itself is stressful and takes an emotional and psychological toll on those who do it. For me, listening to men's misogyny, and at the same time their dependence on women, has on occasion made me feel despair. Sometimes I can find nothing worthy in men and male culture at all. Hearing women's forgiveness, and their hope and encouragement, is often what has kept me going. On occasion too, I have listened to women's insight about their partners' behaviour and wondered why we need sociological accounts at all. On the whole, I find now that I like women more and men less.

Spending so much time with men questioning their attitudes, beliefs and behaviour means that I constantly question my own. I have learned a great deal about myself, and indeed about my own ability to be abusive. I am more alert to the impact my behaviour has on others, and much more conscious generally of how I behave.

Positives

The reader may be forgiven for thinking by now that the work has little to recommend it, but it does have positive aspects. There are some rewards on a regular basis. Many men have a real commitment to the work. Some are aware of the damage and pain they have inflicted on their partners and actively want to change. Some work very hard in the group and and seeing them make progress is very heartening. This can happen at different stages for different men. For some there are real moments of revelation. At times it seems as if a light-bulb comes on in a man's head as some aspect of the work comes home to him. Sessions where this kind of dawning of enlightenment takes place help rekindle my enthusiasm for the task.

The main reward is that I believe I have seen that men *can* change. Listening to some of them talk with wonder and enthusiasm about the difference the programme has made to their lives, and much more importantly hearing women confirm that their partners have changed for the better, more than compensates for the difficulties and stresses involved.

NOTES

1 The CHANGE Project is based in Central Region in Scotland. The Project is funded by the Urban Programme under the sponsorship of Central Region Social Work Department.
2 Generally, the policy of CHANGE is not to accept men who have severe drinking or drug problems.
3 These definitions are reminiscent of Segal's comments 'to be masculine is *not* to be feminine, *not* to be gay, *not* to be tainted with any marks of inferiority – ethnic or otherwise' (1990a: xi).

Chapter 4

Challenges in working with male social work students

Siobhan Lloyd and Dorothy Degenhardt

The context in which men are trained to be social work practitioners has undergone a number of changes in recent years. The
changing emphases on qualifying courses, the introduction of the
Diploma in Social Work and the framework for education and
training outlined in Paper 30 (CCETSW 1989) have all played
an important part. Of course social work training does not take
place in an educational vacuum and students are faced in their
placements with the changing priorities in practice and the consequences of political and economic change. This chapter focuses
on issues relating to male students in training. It starts with a
brief summary of the authors' own experience as social work
educators and trainers and moves on to examine a theoretical
framework which offers a context in which male students can
locate their learning. It examines some implications of the gender
balance in educational institutions and assesses the way ahead
for working with men in social work education.

In writing the chapter we start with an acknowledgement of
the feminist writers who have focused their energy primarily
on the experience of women; we have used their thinking and
writing as an inital focus for our own work (Hudson 1985;
Hanmer and Statham 1988; Dominelli and McLeod 1989; Langan
and Day 1993; Phillipson 1992). With few exceptions, however,
male social work educators and trainers have done little to
develop the many insights afforded by a feminist analysis of
power, gender and care work (Bowl 1985; Abramovitz 1987;
Harper 1987; Ruxton 1992). Using our collective experiences in
social work education and training we make some suggestions
about ways in which male and female educators can work with

male students in addressing gender issues and sexism within a social work context.

Siobhan: Between 1979 and 1990 I taught on social work courses in two Scottish universities. I arrived as a young lecturer, straight from practice as a community worker in Liverpool and with a personal history which allowed me to identify myself as a white, middle-class Irishwoman. I had discovered feminism as a student in Ireland in the early 1970s and, when I came to social work education, this was the strand of my identity which was to become most important in both my professional and personal life. At that time there was no discussion of gender issues on the first course on which I taught. I was nervous enough about my role as a 'serious' academic having just come from practice as a community worker, never mind having the confidence to raise gender issues as a valid part of the curriculum in college and in placements. When I think about it now, I am aware that what I tried to do was to introduce it all by subterfuge – offering options on topics such as 'Working with Women in the Community' or 'Violence in the Family'. This was in a department without overt sexism and in a supportive staff group where six of us held a wide range of perspectives on the nature of social work. In 1989 I started to teach on an undergraduate course in Women's Studies and the experience of this course, in which feminism was the overtly stated theoretical perspective, gave me the confidence to become more explicit in my social work teaching. For example, in the teaching of social policy I used feminism as one of a number of theoretical perspectives with which to understand social problems and was helped in this by the development of a literature with a feminist perspective (Ungerson 1985; Pascall 1986; Glendinning and Millar 1987). As an activist in the women's movement it was also possible to bring a feminist perspective into teaching on violence against women and children. Another significant milestone was contributing to and attending CCETSW's Gender Conferences, held annually for women in social work education and training in Scotland, between 1990 and 1993.

I left social work education as the first students on the Diploma in Social Work were completing their first year and am not, therefore, in a position to comment in any detailed way in which issues relating to the training of male social workers have been developed on these courses. In twelve years' teaching in social work, however, it has been possible to note some positive trends and, certainly, some areas where the work could be further developed. For example, there is now a much greater willingness to place and develop gender on the education and training agenda, albeit from the perspective of working with women as colleagues and clients rather than in relation to men reassessing their values and attitudes; a framework for such work, outlined in CCETSW'S Paper 30, recently revised; more innovative methods for teaching in this area; a growing feminist literature which has gradually ensured that gender issues can no longer be marginalised or be labelled as a 'fringe' concern. This has been due to the sustained and challenging work of feminists within social work education and its related disciplines, the women's movement and the voice of female consumers of social work services.

Alongside these positive developments there are a number of persistent blocks which make advances less easy to confirm. These include a lack of knowledge and training for trainers and educators themselves on what the core issues are and how to go about imparting them to students; persistent questioning from colleagues, both male and, less frequently, female, about the validity of the work; continued undermining of women who are explicit in their commitment to gender issues by labelling them 'trouble-makers'; an assumption that it will be women students and educators who raise the issue, allowing men to remain at best reactive or, at worst, unwilling participants in the process of change.

Dorothy: I have worked with social work students as a practice teacher since the mid-1970s and since 1990 as a social work tutor. It was only after travelling in Asia in the late 1970s and observing the more obvious inequalities for women that my emerging feminist views made me question the sexism in my own country and in my chosen profession. Being involved in social work education and training over the last decade has helped me move from the questioning of structural oppression to thinking about the ways in which we work with male students in considering gender issues and sexism in social work.

As a tutor working with students on the first Diploma in Social Work programme in my college in 1990, I was involved in planning a curriculum which attempts to teach anti-discriminatory practice, including gender issues, both in discrete slots and integrated into all subjects using CCETSW's Paper 30 Requirements (CCETSW 1989) as a framework. I have also been involved in the training of practice teachers, following CCETSW's Paper 26.3 and, while training social workers on the anti-discriminatory practice module, I have encouraged them to consider anti-sexist practice and power/gender issues in their supervision with students in practice.

More specifically, I have tutored women and men in student groups. I have observed that a lower proportion of men is accepted onto our social work course and that men have a higher drop-out rate than female students. This has implications for management of the course in general, and of the tutorial group in particular, where there may only be one male student present. I have also been involved in assertiveness training as part of the training for 'managing difficult or challenging situations'. I have worked with some success with both mixed and single-sex groups. The single-sex group has given group members support in their communality of expression and behaviour, but has not always allowed them to express their differences. The creation of a safe learning environment is ultimately dependent on more than just the gender of the students concerned.

Within teaching sessions on work with older adults, I have noticed that the attention of male students heightens as they realise that social work is not just about caring for older adults but, in the light of community care policies, that there is more emphasis on policy decisions, management of resources and higher-status posts.

The emphasis on anti-discriminatory practice within Paper 30 has enabled anti-sexism to be taken more seriously. However, there seems to be a general expectation that it is women who will initiate training on anti-sexist practice, and these women educators may then find their work undermined and undervalued. The Gender Conferences organised by CCETSW in Scotland since 1990 for women in social work and training have greatly assisted in developing and supporting women educators, and have given me more confidence to pursue these issues.

THE SEARCH FOR A FRAMEWORK

It has been suggested that, throughout the 1970s and 1980s, more women who were active in the women's movement, or who had at least been influenced by the basic tenets of feminism entered social work training (Hudson 1985, 1989). It followed therefore that their experience as social workers would be influenced by some measure of critical understanding about the complicated interface between gender relations and the state. The extent to which ·this has been the case is not yet clear, being dependent on the value-base of courses which the women undertook, the theoretical perspective of their educators and the opportunities for developing their understanding which were presented by their placements.

If we accept that feminism has informed social work to some extent, we may also need to accept that one of its limitations may have been to reduce issues about gender to 'working with women' (Hudson 1992: 78). This is not to imply, however, that movement has been negligible or that there will be no further development. Indeed, as our own biographies have indicated, there have been significant positive changes in the extent to which gender issues have a place in social work education and training.

The framework for working on gender issues is limited because social work educators and trainers, whether or not they identify themselves as feminist, do not consistently state the significance of feminism as a theoretical framework which can inform social work practice. It may be implicit, but this standpoint can devalue its significance and assure a 'safer' approach. It is embodied in using terms such as 'non-sexist' or 'women-centred' rather than 'feminist', possibly because of the anticipated negative effects of being labelled feminist. A number of consequences arise out of this:

* Practice is often atheoretical and, by implication, uncritical of the context in which it takes place and the methods which it uses. As a result it can become too task-centred.
* Feminist theory runs the risk of becoming marginalised within the established canon of social work theory, in which psycho-dynamic perspectives are being replaced by an ascendency of new management theory. This must be understood against the backdrop of an anti-feminist backlash (Faludi 1992).
* There is potential for social work practice theory to be applied

in a highly discriminatory way. MacLeod and Saraga (1988) provide evidence for this in relation to family therapy and systems theory in working with families where there are suspicions of child sexual abuse.

- Men (clients and social workers) are placed at the periphery in terms of challenging their own assumptions, value-base and practice. We believe that the theoretical framework which has been of such value *to* women and in working *with* women, has much to offer men as students, educators, trainers and clients.

Phillipson offers a useful starting point when she argues that feminism as a theoretical framework can be used 'to enable men to see what has to be done, to encourage them to do it and to suggest some ways forward' (1992: 9). She describes how social work has pathologised women or rendered them invisible when, by the same token, men have been 'largely absent from critical consideration, whether as policy-makers, workers or recipients of services' (1992: 21). Segal develops this view, suggesting that men must start to 'acknowledge their need to change, to abandon a masculinity which is destructive both towards women and towards their own nature' (1990a: 61). She argues that it is men's generalised fear of intimacy which has held them in a state of isolation and fear from one another and from women and that this, in part, offers an explanation for their violence towards one another and towards women.

Phillipson advocates that the first step in developing a feminist theoretical framework for social work education is the adoption of a 'gender lens', which allows the individual or group the opportunity to 'look at the familiar from a different perspective' (1992: 27). She takes this idea further, suggesting that there are two prior stages for arriving at a model for feminist practice. The first stage centres on the development of a universal anti-oppressive practice, which might also include anti-ageist, anti-disablist, anti-homophobic and anti-racist practice, and the second moves on to a specifically anti-sexist practice. Only then is it possible to work towards a form of social work practice which is feminist in nature.

Four themes from the women's movement might usefully be adopted by male students for a feminist analysis in social work.

The personal is political

Just as the slogan became a powerful public statement of the way in which experiences and problems of individual women have historical, economic and cultural dimensions, men can be encouraged to use this as a means of reflecting on their own lives and experience.

Standpoint theory

It is argued that women occupy a privileged standpoint which gives them access not only to the world of their own lives, but also to that of the dominant, male group through women's greater awareness of the complexities of social life and the socially constructed nature of the world. Although standpoint theory has been criticised because it does not fully acknowledge the diversity between women and because it ignores the question of masculinities (Longino 1993), it can challenge phallocentric views of the world and help to eliminate the false distinction between the public and private domain. Standpoint theory provides a useful framework for locating the dual roles of women, their fractured identities and the socially constructed expectations of them as carers. The application of standpoint theory for men lies in its ability to validate these fractured identities; men too might be encouraged to think of the ways in which their experience is fragmented and the effects of this on their ability to be emotional and to connect with others, in both their personal and professional lives. Male social workers in training could therefore be encouraged to immerse themselves in feminist literature on a particular topic or hear, first hand, from women about the nature of their experience as women in a patriarchal world. As Cain eloquently puts it:

If you want to know *for* women, you must organically connect yourself *with* women, move to an appropriate site from which to generate this knowledge. Both men and women can and have to do this. Goodwill is not enough. Being a woman does not mean that one can automatically speak for women from a feminist standpoint.

(1986: 132)

A study of masculinity

There is scope for an examination of the nature of masculinity itself, much in the same way as the social construction of femininity has been analysed and challenged by feminism (Archer and Lloyd 1985; Eichenbaum and Orbach 1985; Oakley 1985; Brownmiller 1986; Dworkin 1988). It has been pointed out, however, that many feminists equate masculinity with male dominance and, according to this view, the psychology of men inevitably perpetuates the social structures of male dominance as a result of the features of either biological or social construction (Segal 1990a). Other writers distinguish masculinity and male dominance while accepting the existence of connections between the psychology of men and the social structures of male dominance (Chodorow 1980; Pleck 1981; Eichenbaum and Orbach 1985). This approach has led to an exploration of the experience and subjectivity of men in more detail. Some attempt has been made by men themselves in sections of the 'men's movement' to assert men's capacity to transform their behaviour so that it is more egalitarian. However, some men in the movement have focused on a reassertion of masculinity by restoring men's primitive instincts and enjoyment of their masculinity, embodied in the 'wild man within' (Bly 1991). There is also the suggestion that if men wish to assert themselves as individuals they should take back the power they have given to women in the role of mother (Faludi 1992). This is hardly in tune with a feminist analysis and indeed, there are some writers who align themselves with this movement who are openly hostile to feminism (Lyndon 1992; Thomas 1993).

Theory and experience

The grounding of theory in experience has been a major contribution of the women's movement (Roberts 1981; McLeod 1987; Stanley and Wise 1993). Carter et al. (1992) have stressed that it is only by making sense of everyday experience that a theoretical framework can be constructed. For men in social work this means, for example, examining the ways in which they and other men arrive at social work roles which demand a degree of regulating or controlling. It can extend to an examination of similar processes operating inside social work education which can place women in caring roles, leaving men to control and manage. Although the care/control dichotomy can be an issue for both women and men in social work, there is always the risk that men may be more attracted to practice placements which are more concerned with control aspects of social work, an issue explored further later in this chapter. Even the process of the student's entry into social work education, their role models in the training institution and in social work practice can be used to construct a framework for understanding.

All of this suggests that a feminist conceptual framework offers a sound basis for analysing both male and female experience and that it also offers optimistic prospects for change. For male social workers in training it offers the chance to analyse critically their own theoretical perspective, to enrich their learning and, ultimately, to increase their understanding of practice. These are all themes which we have found particularly useful, not only in our understanding of the world in which we live, but in our work with men in the field of social work education and training. It is appropriate at this point, therefore, to examine that context more closely. Who are the men in social work training, both students and trainers/educators, and how can we work with them in more constructive ways?

WHERE ARE THE MEN IN SOCIAL WORK EDUCATION AND TRAINING?

There are two main areas to consider in answering this question. First, there are issues which relate to the role models of men and women who are social work educators and trainers, their role and status within teaching groups, the subjects on which they teach and research and the methods which they use. Second, there are issues relating to men as student social workers. These include their experience in college and on placement and the extent to which their placements are an indication of future career destinations. There are also important issues relating to the way in which men are made aware of the significance of gender on social work courses and how this material is taught.

The social work learning environment

Students are influenced in all sorts of ways by their training environment – the way in which teaching is conducted, curriculum content, their peer group and the ways in which a course enables them to reflect on their personal and professional development. The role models presented by their educators and trainers offers another source of learning and there are significant gender issues here. Women currently occupy only 18 per cent of tenured academic posts in the United Kingdom (Caplan 1993). Table 4.1 shows the national situation in Scotland, where women make up 21 per cent of academic staff overall (Scottish Office 1992).

Table 4.1 Representation of women in Scottish universities in 1991

Academic posts	Women in post	Women as % of total
Professors	31	4
Senior lecturers	141	9
Lecturers	990	24
Other academic staff	482	47

Source: Scottish Office (1992) Statistical Bulletin, Education Series, Edinburgh

The largest number of women are in untenured and short-term appointments. The picture is one of an 'academic funnel', with large numbers of female students gradually narrowing down to a small number of tenured female academic staff and, inevitably, an even smaller number of senior women academics (Abramovitz 1985). Table 4.2, which provides a snapshot of social work teaching staff in Scottish higher education in 1994, displays a more complicated picture.

There are a number of interesting contradictions presented in the table. Women are well-represented at professorial/head of department level, where two of the four appointments have been made within the last two years. Women are under-represented at senior lecturer level, confirming the national trend within higher education, and well represented at basic lecturer grade. Unsurprisingly, the majority of part-time lecturers are female.There is also some limited evidence to suggest that female social work academics are less active in research and writing than their male counterparts (Kirk and Rosenblatt 1984; Abramovitz 1985).

Our own experience would suggest that students can quickly become aware of a gender division in academia which is perpetu-

Table 4.2 Representation of women in social work teaching in Scottish universities and colleges, June 1994

	Professor/ Head of Department	Senior Lecturer	Lecturer	Part-time Lecturer
Colleges				
Female	1	2	15	2
Male	2	4	9	1
Universities				
Female	4	0	11	11
Male	2	6	8	2
Total	9	12	43	16
Women as % of total	55	16	60	81

Source: Personal communication with educational institutions

ated by the education system in a number of ways. These include teaching responsibilities which might emphasise a theory (male)/ practice (female) split, and teaching styles and reading lists which do not maintain a gender balance. Although gender differences in teaching style on social work courses have not been researched in a systematic way, we have observed a greater willingness by female educators and trainers to balance didactic teaching with experiential learning methods (Crawley 1983; Brady 1989). This issue is emphasised by Bailey and Cox (1993) in their analysis of teaching styles on a social work course. They note the way in which experiential teaching was positively evaluated by female staff, whereas male tutors argued that such methods perpetuated an anti-intellectual stance within social work. This links with the conceptual framework outlined at the start of this chapter which stresses the importance of using experience as the starting point from which a theory can be constructed.

A further dimension to the role models offered to female and male students relates to collaborative and team teaching. Kearney and Le Riche (1993), describing their experience of teaching gender issues on a postgraduate child protection course, noted the male devaluing of joint working in teaching social work practice and management. Whilst they do not offer any reasons for men working less frequently in this way, they point out that female staff are open to working collaboratively for a number of reasons including mutual support, peer review and a commitment to a more open model of teaching. Phillipson (1993) develops this point in a discussion of female management styles when she asserts that women's caring role and, consequently, their power, often signifies an attempt to interact with other people in ways that further the development of other people, empowering them and building up their strength and resources, effectiveness and well-being. There is, of course, a down-side to this in both practice and teaching contexts, since women's willingness to nurture and care can reinforce men's expectations of being cared for which in turn reinforce women in a caring role, thus enabling men to retain their power.

Our experience has been that we have both undertaken a greater proportion of team teaching with female colleagues, even when there have been more men in the staff group. We have also observed that male colleagues are less likely to initiate ideas for team teaching and, when they do, female colleagues are frequently cast in the role of 'supporting cast' rather than as equal partners in the venture. This presents women with the dilemma of continually challenging the assumptions of male colleagues or being perceived by students as an unequal partner in the teaching programme. These choices are not easily or consistently made. From our own experience one way ahead was to raise the issue in a staff meeting not as a problem area but within the context of establishing a code of practice for joint teaching ventures. This had the added advantage of allowing future team teaching to be openly evaluated.

Another strand in this discussion relates to the way in which women and men communicate with each other and with students. Lakoff (1975) developed this work in an analysis of female and male speech patterns which started with the proposition that men's language is one of domination, whilst women's language is tentative. Carli (1990) has taken the work forward by looking at speech forms adapted to different contexts rather than one-off speech events. She shows how women are more tentative in their speech when they are paired with men, using more hesitant, qualifying or apologetic phrases. Tannen (1992), building on Gilligan's work (1982), takes a slightly different approach, arguing that women's speech patterns demonstrate a search for intimacy whilst those of men are more conscious of status and adversarial roles. She argues that when sympathy and concern are expressed, they are interpreted by women as signifying understanding and searching for symmetry between equals, whereas for men they signify an expression of weakness and condescension. She suggests that men have a need to appear skilful and knowledgeable whilst maintaining connections with others, whereas for women it is more important to seek support and cohesiveness. Our own experience would confirm this pattern to some extent, and it has made us review the way in which our personal styles might be more rigorous and challenging when working with groups.

What consequences does this have for the teaching styles of male and female tutors and for the context in which the learning takes place? It has implications for working in single-sex groups, for example, where male staff members can be encouraged to support one another and to model skills for encouraging students to do likewise. We would also argue from our experience, however, that some men cannot be trusted with this work and that same-gender male tutor pairs can lead to collusion, with denial and avoidance of difficult issues. One way of improving teaching styles would be for women to work more closely with their male counterparts on gender training, offering students a role model, and being as open as possible about any difficulties which may arise in the process. This would also enable female tutors to set the agenda in a way which addresses key issues without compromise or an abuse of power. It would be questionable, however, how far male tutors were genuinely intent on co-working in an egalitarian way, rather than engaging in the enterprise simply because it was a requirement of the course.

Issues in working with the student group

The dynamic of the student group is a powerful force in teaching and, faced with the prospect of presenting a feminist perspective on an issue, a female staff member can feel isolated and vulnerable. Male students can be defensive if this is new material to them, and their response can be to minimise, to excuse or, at worst, to deny its validity. In addition, female students, fearful of attack for expressing feminist views, may show sympathy to their male peers. The lecturer/tutor has then to make choices about whether to talk the men through the issues in the group or to leave it with them. She needs also to consider how to explain to the women in the group the notion of this 'sympathy trap' which absolves men from taking responsibility for the behaviour of their gender.

Dealing with male defensiveness once it has been identified is not easy. It might include doing the teaching in mixed or single-sex pairs or devising strategies which will allow the women and men in the group to express their views in a less personally threatening way. This can be done by using scenarios or vignettes rather than asking students to use their own experience, thus giving students the choice of talking about personal experience in a supportive or 'disguised' way.

In most educational or training contexts there are some students who monopolise discussion and others who remain silent. There are men who refuse to engage in any discussion of gender issues and those who take over women's space in an exploitative way. In the former case, one response might be quickly to divide the group into single-sex pairs, setting them a short task which they are then asked to discuss with a 'pair' of the other sex. The same tactic can be employed in the second situation, this time making the groups larger and, when they join, nominating an observer to plot the contributions based on gender. A useful follow-up would be to give a short presentation on the gender language features in group discussion based on Carli's (1990) work.

Our own experience confirms that it is impossible to plan for every eventuality but that, when faced with either of the two common situations outlined above, 'time out' in a single-sex group has a number of significant advantages in moving a difficult situation on. First, it takes the pressure off those who might be finding the situation increasingly uncomfortable; second, it challenges students to be accountable to their own gender group, and third, it allows the students to see that tutors can empower students by giving them responsibility for their own learning.

An important consideration in all of this is to acknowledge that as women we present a role model for all students. Women students will watch how we respond to male colleagues and may be able to learn from this. Of course they too have much to teach their tutors and one another. In many ways, therefore, the identification of strategies for working with men aims to strive for change in men and to enable women to identify useful strategies in their interaction with men.

Men as students

Recent figures suggest that during the 1980s there was a steady decline in the number of men entering social work (La Valle and Lyons 1993). The percentage of men who qualified as social workers also declined during this period, from 38 per cent in 1983 to 25 per cent in 1991 (CCETSW, quoted in La Valle and Lyons 1993). In one Scottish Diploma in Social Work course, the non-completion rate for men between 1991 and 1993 was between 30 and 50 per cent, whilst for women it was between 10 and 20 per cent (personal communication 1994). Given that there are fewer applications from men in the first place, the male non-completion rate on social work courses has a number of potential consequences, including: the ways in which the remaining men are treated as a minority group; the implications of having single-sex groups for men on courses when there may not be enough men to form a reasonably sized group; and the interaction between male and female tutors and male students who are in the minority.

There is little information about the post-qualifying destinations of students, or about their subsequent career paths. It has been suggested, however, that social work education has helped to perpetuate occupational segregation patterns in which women, black and working-class people are disproportionately concentrated in lower-status and less well-paid jobs (Howe 1986). In addition, the changing nature of social work education looks as though it will reinforce this pattern as more women workers in the caring role are guided to NVQ/SVQ and HNC training rather than the apparently more 'professional' Diploma in Social Work and later post-qualifying training. There is already some evidence that child protection work, formerly a female ghetto, has become a 'desirable' destination for the aspiring male manager (Hudson 1992). This is beginning to be echoed in the field of community care with its resource management culture.

Placement choice

One of the possible indicators of change is the choice which students make for their final placement, or Area of Particular Practice. This placement is used as a guide to the area of work in which the qualified worker aims to practise. The choice of

Area of Particular Practice is, of course, affected by placement availability and the competition for placements between courses and within student groups. Table 4.3 gives an indication of the spread of these placements in Scotland in 1994.

The data presented in this table should be considered within the overall contexts of larger numbers of female social work students in training than male and the limitations on availability and choice of placements for students. Although it is too early to draw firm conclusions, we may be witnessing the start of a trend for men towards community care placements. One proposition, that community care may offer a potential career path, merits further investigation. Similarly, the fact that women are still over-represented in placements which focus on children suggests that women continue to see where their careers within social work lie (Howe 1986).

There are also some interesting geographical differences shown in the tables. For example, Northern Consortium has a larger percentage of men working in childcare placements than in other regions and proportionately fewer men in community care placements. This, however, may reflect the availability of placements rather than a positive choice on their part for practice in the childcare arena.

SOME WAYS AHEAD

If social work educators and trainers are committed to developing anti-sexist social work practice there are a number of key issues which need to be addressed. First, as we have already indicated, it is vital that there is an overt commitment to the inclusion of feminism as a valid theoretical framework. This would allow both female and male students to address their current practice critically and to make clearer links between their public and private lives. It would also ensure that feminism becomes part of the mainstream of social work theory.

Second, the building of alliances between women and men could be developed. Gay men, older men, men from minority ethnic groups and men with disabilities all face oppression in society, and exploration of forms and experiences of oppression shared with women would be useful. In this respect, however, attention needs to be paid to the potentially negative consequences of constructing alliances which focus exclusively on a

Table 4.3 Areas of Particular Practice placements across three Scottish consortia: 1992–94 intake (1)

	Northern (2)				Lothian and Borders				Tayforth			
	Children/ Families	Community care	Criminal justice	Total	Children/ Families	Community care	Criminal justice	Total	Children/ Families	Community care	Criminal justice	Total
Female	16(39)	17(41)	8(19)	41(100)	31(51)	23(38)	7(11)	61(100)	14(67)	4(19)	3(14)	21(100)
Male	9(56)	5(31)	2(12)	16(100)	6(26)	13(57)	4(17)	23(100)	2(50)	1(25)	1(25)	3(100)

Notes:
Figures in brackets represent percentage of total placements in each category.

(1) Two courses do not operate these types or placements.
(2) A further 6 students undertook generic field social work placements in this consortium area.

Source: Personal communication with colleges and universities

shared oppression. The recognition of diversity is as important as the sharing of common experience for both women and men in any area of their lives. This point is developed by Stanley (1982), who indicates the inherent dangers in assuming that the gay men's movement and the women's movement have the same perspective on the oppression of gay men and lesbians, and she warns against a common grouping.

Third, there is the related issue of the potential for men to learn from one another. Creating opportunities for them to work in single-sex groups in college and on placement on issues relating to masculinity might help to ensure that they confront the sources of their own oppression and oppressive practices. The question of whether men can be relied upon to carry this through may need to be set against the responsibility of women becoming more proactive in working alongside men in the change process. Phillipson (1992) again offers some useful ideas. She advocates the application of Friere's framework of 'perspective transformation' which encourages the questioning of previously held beliefs about roles by trying out different ways of seeing and behaving (Friere 1972). This perspective offers men a way to unlearn, reframe and change when they are faced with traditional expectations of masculinity. In the final analysis the most appropriate response may rest on the stage in the process at which women and men are sited (Humphries 1989).

Fourth, an emphasis on training for care rather than control is vital in the context of men's future destination as social workers. The timing of these changes may be politically difficult as the climate for innovation in social work education and training is changing, with an increasing emphasis on functional analysis rather than on training for care. Social work educators and trainers still have a responsibility, however, to include interpersonal skills on the training agenda for all students.

Fifth, anti-racist training has some useful insights to offer in terms of understanding a perspective of oppression which has not been directly experienced (Boushel 1991). Skills used in training white students to understand black people's oppression could be transferred into anti-sexist training so that men can understand women's oppression. Anti-racist training has attempted to develop the means to enable students to challenge their own racism; it is valid to build on this experience when students share their experiences in single-sex groups.

There are a number of simple ways in which these recommendations for developing an anti-sexist approach to social work teaching could be incorporated into the social work curriculum as it presently stands. They include:

- bringing in outside trainers, especially for work in single-sex groups – note that the question of accountability would need to be decided (that is, how much men are expected to report back to women on their work);
- developing placement opportunities which assess men in a more overtly caring role;
- redesigning existing courses so that the developing feminist literature in the fields of sociology, psychology, law, social policy, working with families and with young people, for example, is integral;
- developing assessment criteria which will test the competencies of male students actively to address issues relating to gender in their training and practice;
- the training of educators and practice teachers in gender issues so that they can be encouraged to provide role models in anti-oppressive teaching and practice for both their female and male students.

The final word rests with a reworking of Freud's famous question, as developed by Segal:

> What is it that men want? If only they could tell us. If only they could communicate their feelings. Throughout history we, who are women, have knocked our heads against the riddle, have been begging men on our knees, and still cannot learn from them why they present to us such sinister contrasts – the baby and the bully, the rapist and the romantic, the hard and the soft, the terrifying and the ridiculous. Those of you who are men have escaped worrying about this problem – you are yourselves the problem.
>
> (1990a: 61)

Chapter 5

Why do men care?

Viviene E. Cree

This chapter will examine new research into men and professional social work. This research, which seeks to discover why men choose to enter professional social work training, contributes to a wider feminist enquiry into women and caring, and specifically addresses the question 'Why do *men* care?'

The chapter is organised in three broad sections. The first section discusses how I came to be interested in a study of men, and describes my journey from work with women and research into women's lives into a new awareness of the need for a greater understanding of the position of men in social work. The second section outlines the research I have conducted with men and women first-year social work students. The last section draws out the main themes from the research, and asks what the implications are for women and for men in terms of reaching a new feminist perspective on gender differences in social work and in caring.

BACKGROUND

The major part of my personal and professional life to date has been spent with women. I grew up the middle daughter of three girls and spent much of my childhood in conventional girls' activities – Brownies, Girl Guides, helping at home and playing 'housies' and 'schoolies' with my sisters and any neighbourhood children we could draw into our games. As a student in the early 1970s I embraced the women's liberation movement for the first time, and was able to reconcile my personal experiences with a political reality and a set of strategic objectives. Trips on minibuses to London to join National Abortion Campaign demonstrations, local campaigning for a women's health centre, self-examination and consciousness-raising were as fundamental to my university experience as any study of Middle English or Moral Philosophy. After a post-graduate Diploma, I worked for sixteen years as a social worker, choosing to work in situations where I could maximise my commitment to women – girls' groups, pregnancy counselling, groups for lone parents (mothers), community work with women and children, practice teaching. I am now teaching social work students, 70 per cent of whom are women (Central Council for Education and Training in Social Work figures for Scotland, 1993–94).

I have not, of course, inhabited a world made up only of women. My father, various male teachers and a succession of boyfriends had a huge impact on my life and on my view of myself. But my greatest energies were put towards working with women, and with the exception of the man who became my partner, I chose (along with many other feminists of my generation) to leave men to get on with their own affairs. My position on this has now changed dramatically. I believe that it is vital that we engage with men – to challenge men, to support men, to *change* men – and that this is essential if there is to be any real change in society for women and men.

My attitude shift has come about for a mixture of reasons, again personal and professional. I am now the mother of two sons, and have been able to see at first hand the development of their personalities, and the difficulties they continue to experience growing up as boys (Phillips 1993). I have also experienced at times my imperfections as a mother, and have felt deeply the inadequacy of psychological notions that women have special innate 'caring' qualities (Chodorow 1978).

Personal learning has been matched by experiences in my professional work. In the mid-1980s, a woman colleague and I set up a centre for women and children in a deprived council housing scheme on the outskirts of Edinburgh. Our approach was unapologetically feminist. We sought to build on our shared experience as women: to reduce the power imbalance between ourselves and the women who came to the centre by encouraging member-participation, and by working in as non-hierarchical a way as possible. In reality, the distance between us and the women using the centre was massive. Poverty, social class, poor housing, drug and alcohol abuse, and lack of life choice meant that the differences between us and the centre users were irreconcilable. Just as important, we could not deny our role as social workers, faced as we were at times with overwhelming evidence of child abuse and neglect. We were feminist social workers seeking to empower and support women, yet our job was also to control and set limits on women's parenting, and on occasions, to take children into care. This experience was fundamental for me in terms of developing a realistic, honest, feminist social work practice (Wise 1990).

Another significant step on my professional path was research undertaken for a PhD. In 1989 I began a case-study of Family Care, a voluntary social work agency based in Edinburgh, with its origins in the National Vigilance Association (Cree 1995). I interviewed former social workers and asked them about their work, and specifically about their reasons for coming into social work. Ninety-seven per cent of my respondents were women, many of whom described their work in terms of 'service'. Caring for others came much higher up the agenda for these largely middle-class women than other concerns such as financial remuneration or career advancement. Service to others, and very often, service to God, was totally connected with their view of themselves as women. It was their primary function and reason for being.

This discovery led me to explore literature around women and caring – psychological studies which suggest that caring for others is fundamental to women's psyche (Baker Miller 1978; Chodorow 1978), and philosophical studies which view women's moral development as radically different from that of men (Gilligan 1982). I was critical of this literature for two reasons: first, because of the harsh judgements which society makes of women who do not live up to this stereotypical picture; and second, because essentialist positions always seem pessimistic about the possibility of change – of greater equality between men and women. Grant offers a third criticism. She writes: 'it is not clear to me why an argument that women are different and better than men is any more sound than one that claims that women are different and inferior' (1993: 63).

This chapter focuses on research which attempts to understand more about the question of caring and women/men. My point of departure is as follows: assuming that women choose to become social workers because caring is somehow central to their sense of self, why do *men* choose to become social workers? Are their reasons for entering professional social work significantly different from those of women? What does this therefore tell us about social work, and about men and women?

RESEARCH QUESTION – WHY SOCIAL WORK?

In the winter of 1993/94, I conducted a research study based on thirty-five male and female students in their first year of social work training at four Diploma in Social Work programmes in Scotland. I invited respondents to tell me in their own words what they believed were the factors and influences which had led them to take up social work as a career, and engaged them in a wide-ranging discussion about their perceptions of social work, and about the place of men and women within social work. I also asked them to complete a questionnaire entitled Occupational Decision Making, in which they placed in rank order motivational factors (such as promotion opportunities, friendship opportunities, flexible working hours and creativity) in choosing social work as a career. Finally, at the end of the interview I carried out a Bem androgyny test on each student. (Examples of both are included in the Appendix to this chapter.)

Theoretical ideas and principles underpinning the research were influenced by my experience as a feminist sociologist working in social work. Feminist sociologists have argued that conventional sociology has ignored women's experience, and has created a set of structures and way of thinking about society which is based on men as the norm. The first objective of feminist sociology was to redress this imbalance, and to begin to explain the world from the perspective of women (Spender 1981; Bell and Roberts 1984; Smith 1987; Maynard 1990; Stanley 1990). There is now a broader sociological agenda, albeit a minority one, which is centred on exploring the gendered lives of both women and men. Here there is a recognition that it is necessary for women to carry out research on men and boys, as part of a bigger project of reformulating sociology (Abbott and Wallace 1990).

Feminist research, however, is about more than the subject under investigation. It is also about the ways in which that study is carried out. As a feminist sociologist, I wished to carry out a study which would be purposeful in feminist terms. It was to be action-based, and rooted in experience (Stanley 1990). It was to have the potential for consciousness-raising, for women and for men (Cook and Fonow 1986). And it was to have meaning for me as a social worker and a social work teacher. I was not an objective 'outsider' adopting a neutral, scientific pose (Mies 1983). Instead I had a strong vested interest in the subject area and in the outcome of the research. The whole existence of the study related to my personal, professional and political history, while the planning and conduct of the research reflected my social work experience and most particularly, my experience of person-centred counselling (Rogers 1951).

RESEARCH METHODS

The sample

My sample group was made up of seventeen men and eighteen women in their first year of Diploma in Social Work training at four academic institutions in Scotland.

All the students were white and of European ethnic origin. The one black student from the Diploma in Social Work programmes with which I was working declined to take part in the research. One-third of the students were on secondment; one was self-funding; and the remainder were on grants from Central Council for Education and Training in Social Work (CCETSW). Students' ages varied considerably, from twenty-three to forty-six years of age. Almost three-quarters of the women whom I interviewed were parents, 70 per cent of whom were lone parents. While 40 per cent of the men were parents, only one was a lone parent caring for a child.

Although my sample of respondents was relatively small, I am confident (from my experience in practice teaching and lecturing in social work) that the students whom I met were broadly typical of social work students in their first year of training in Scotland. Figures produced annually by CCETSW place my study in a Scottish-wide context. Of those 471 students beginning social work training in Scotland in 1993, 137 were men (29 per cent), and 334 were women (71 per cent). Only 16 (3.4 per cent) of the students gave their racial origin as black or other; 455 (96.6 per cent) described themselves as white. Figures indicate that secondments from employers are given to disproportionately high numbers of men. Although secondments were awarded to only

20 per cent of the student population, over 40 per cent of second-ments were given to men, who make up less than 30 per cent of the total student group (CCETSW figures for Scotland, 1993–94).

Individual interviews

I interviewed two male students in the early stages of the research as an exploration of the subject and a pilot of the interview schedule. I then carried out interviews with ten men and fifteen women from three social work programmes (post-qualifying, degree and Diploma courses).

All interviews were tape-recorded. I devised a set of core questions which I put to all respondents, starting with a question about significant life events or experiences which respondents believed had led them to become social workers, and moving to more general questions about the social work task and the place of women and men in social work. Within the confines of the interview, I encouraged respondents to talk to me as freely as possible about whatever aspect of our discussion was most important to them (Bertaux 1981; Oakley 1985; Stanley and Wise 1983; Thompson 1988).

Group interviews

Group interviews performed a different function from those of individual interviews, and were carried out differently. Two single-sex interviews were conducted with five men and three women first-year students at my own academic institution, the University of Edinburgh. I already knew the students from a teaching context, and had built up a measure of mutual trust and respect with them. For ethical reasons, I did not ask the students to give me personal information or details, or to complete questionnaires or androgyny tests. Instead, drawing on Denzin's triangulation method (Denzin 1970), I used the group interviews as a vehicle for checking out themes which emerged in the individual interviews, and for discussing in a more general way the students' views on men and women in social work.

Gender and power in the interview process

I am aware that my gender will have had an impact on the research results (McKee and O'Brien 1983; Finch 1984). Some women may have found it easy to talk to me as a woman, while others may have been suspicious about what they perceived to be my feminist perspective, and felt threatened by my questions. Some men may have felt defensive about the subject-matter of the interviews. I sought to counter-balance the influence of gender by working to put respondents at their ease in the interviews, and by giving them as much control as possible over the research process. By briefing respondents adequately before an interview and by conducting interviews in the form of a dialogue rather than a straight question-and-answer session, I sought to make respondents feel part of the interview process, rather than as if they were objects under investigation (Stanley and Wise 1983).

This does not, of course, imply that dialogue was ever totally reciprocal, or that the interviewer–respondent power imbalance was removed. I was not only a woman interviewing women and men; I was a social work lecturer, and as such, I inevitably held a degree of power over the respondents, even though I did not have involvement in their individual social work courses. I could do little to mitigate this, except to reassure the students that I had no formal contact with their course leaders or tutors. I also chose to use my home address when writing to students to arrange interviews, as a way of reducing social distance between them and me.

Occupational decision-making questionnaire

The twenty-five students who were interviewed on an individual basis completed a questionnaire designed to test how important they regarded various aspects related to their career choice. The students were invited to rate on a scale of 1 to 7 the importance they attached to items as varied as income and pension fund on the one hand and friendship opportunities and personal fulfilment on the other (see Appendix).

The questionnaires, in allowing me to quantify factors, provided an extremely useful counter-balance to the highly personal pictures which emerged in the interviews. They also gave me the opportunity to examine individual features such as importance

given to promotion opportunities, as well as more general categories such as career-based reasons for coming into social work as
opposed to other types of reasons (Bryman 1988; Brannen 1992).

Bem Sex-Role Inventory

The Bem Sex-Role Inventory (BSRI) was developed by Sandra
Bem in the United States in the 1970s as a challenge to traditional
categories of masculine and feminine. Bem argued that masculinity and femininity were two independent dimensions, rather
than opposite ends of a single dimension; men and women could
therefore see themselves as both masculine and feminine (Bem
1974). She developed the BSRI test in which individuals are
asked to locate themselves on a scale of 1 to 7 in terms of twenty
adjectives describing commonly perceived masculine characteristics (for example, ambitious, independent, assertive), twenty
adjectives describing feminine characteristics (for example, affec-
tionate, gentle, understanding), and twenty neutral adjectives (for
example, truthful, happy, conceited) (see Appendix).

The average or mean number of points assigned by each person
to the masculinity attributes constitutes his or her Masculinity
score; the average or mean number of points assigned by each
person to the femininity attributes constitutes his or her Femininity score. Using the median masculinity and femininity scores as
the cut-off points, the person is then classified as either masculine
(high masculine/low feminine), feminine (high feminine/low
masculine), and androgynous (high masculine/high feminine) or
undifferentiated (low masculine/low feminine). Bem's own study
of psychology students at Stanford University in 1975 found that
over one-third of the males and females were 'sex-typed' (masculine men and feminine women); approximately one-quarter
described themselves as either androgynous or undifferentiated;

Table 5.1 BSRI classification of scores

		Masculinity score	
		Below median	*Above median*
Femininity score	Below median	Undifferentiated	Masculine
	Above median	Feminine	Androgynous

and fewer than one-fifth described themselves as 'sex-reversed' (Bem 1977).

I was sceptical about the BSRI for a number of reasons. How valid was its measurement likely to be, given the twenty years which had passed since its inception, and given the cultural and age differences between my own, largely Scottish, sample, and Bem's Stanford University undergraduate student sample? And how does what people say about themselves actually relate to what they do in practice? Hochschild's research into the 'second shift' of childcare and housework indicated that there is often a wide discrepancy between what people *say* they do, and what they actually do at home (Hochschild 1990). Was it possible that my respondents would pick answers which they thought were appropriate for themselves as 'good', 'caring' social work students, rather than where they honestly believed themselves to be? And finally, how useful is such a test in the first place? What does it actually measure? Might its use actually reinforce the very categories of masculine and feminine which I was seeking to challenge?

After much exploration of studies which have used the BSRI (Archer 1989), I finally decided that the BSRI was a useful tool in spite of my misgivings. *Whatever* the BSRI measured, the results would be of interest – simply in terms of seeing if there were similarities and differences in the ways in which men and women scored; and similarities and differences between my sample population and sample populations from other relevant studies.

RESEARCH FINDINGS – MEN AND WOMEN IN SOCIAL WORK

The key finding from my research is that, in spite of the reality that men and women come into social work for many and varied expressed reasons, the career choices and career paths of men and women in social work are significantly affected by issues which are rooted in gendered assumptions and gendered practices. In other words, in spite of individual variations, men and women have different histories and anticipate having different futures within social work.

(a) Reasons for choosing to enter professional social work training

My study indicates that a student's reasons for choosing to enter professional social work training are likely to encompass a range of factors, some related to family background and significant experiences in childhood, and others related to experiences and choices made in adulthood. Some students see social work in career terms only, as a reasonably well-paid job, with good career prospects. Others see it as a vocation, as something to which they have something special to give. While some students may wish to remain in social work, and can map out a path for the years ahead, others have no idea where they will be working in ten years' time, and some do not anticipate being in social work at all.

Family background

There were no significant gender differences in family background separating men and women who entered social work training. The backgrounds of the men and women students whom I interviewed were varied – loving and secure for some students, unsettled and unhappy for others. Some students described a traditional nuclear family upbringing, with father working outside the home and mother's life centred on home and children. Others talked about their mothers' work outside the home, and about growing up with an expectation that household duties would be shared. Some students grew up with one parent after their parents were divorced; another was brought up by grandparents while his parents were working abroad. Almost two-thirds of the total sample came from families with three or more children.

A considerable number of the male students (one-third of the total group) described feeling especially close to their mothers. As one man related, 'I was always sensitive – always attached to my mother' (04M). Another man, whose father spent most of his time working away from home, agreed:

> I was brought up with my mother, two older sisters, my two grans – a lot of female influence. I think this has actually strengthened me, because I have no qualms about emotion, showing my feelings. When I was growing up I took on this macho image which wasn't me – a sort of hard man image –

but deep down inside the true self was there, and would come to the surface occasionally.

(02M)

Other students (men and women) described their fathers as their primary role models – caring people, heavily involved in looking after extended family members, or committed to community activities. Sometimes the motivation for this seems to have been Christian duty; at other times, it was about a socialist principle centred on injustice and inequality, and the need to do something about it; sometimes it was a mixture of both:

My dad worked for British Steel in the furnace. He was one of these people who was always helpful, he always talked to people. I come from a very social family.

(08M)

Research into men in non-traditional settings (as house-husbands, teachers and nurses) suggests that there may be a correlation between men's willingness to take on caring responsibilities and their own experiences of being nurtured by their parents. Some studies have highlighted relationships with mothers as having key significance here (Chusmir 1990). Others have concentrated on the relationship between fathers and sons, arguing on the one hand that sons of absent fathers may wish to compensate by building strong relationships with their own offspring, while on the other hand participative fathers set a good role model for their sons to follow (Rosenwasser and Patterson 1984–85). My study clearly evidences the centrality of parental relationships for male social work students. However, significantly, women students see relationships with parents as equally important.

Significant childhood experiences

An important subject discussed by men and women students was the illness of a parent in childhood. Twenty per cent of the male respondents and almost 50 per cent of the women told me about the impact of the physical or mental illness of a parent. At times this illness was simply described as part of the back-cloth of childhood – a parent was ill, but there was no actual involvement in physical care-giving. At other times, the illness assumed far greater proportions, and dominated the experience of childhood.

Asked to explain what he saw as critical in his decision to become a social worker, a male student related:

> I was told if mum takes a seizure what to do, and I was always praised for that. Being the oldest, it was my responsibility – caring, in a way. I am sure that had a major bearing.
>
> (19M)

Two women and one male student also talked about the death of a parent in childhood. Childhood experiences of illness and loss are noteworthy, especially if they are added to the students whose parents were divorced, and those who were brought up for a time by other relatives. Students describe themselves as sensitised to other people's problems because of their own histories, and wanting to improve systems of caring for the benefit of others. While more women students shared this background, this may simply be a feature of the fact that I carried out more individual interviews with women.

Again, research into men who choose to work in female-dominated settings has suggested that non-traditional men are more likely to have grown up in a lone-parent household, or to have lost a parent or sibling when growing up (Lemkau 1984). This is of note, because parallel research into women in male-dominated occupations indicates that non-traditional women tend to come from a background of family stability and close contact with both a mother and a father (Chusmir 1983). In other words, while some women who enter male worlds may do so from a supportive and secure background, some men who enter female worlds may do so out of instability and disruption.

Two men and one women in my sample described as significant their own experiences of illness and disability, on one occasion necessitating a series of operations in childhood. A man who is registered as blind and has chronic arthritis saw this as a major factor in how he has developed:

> It would be easy to be bitter and angry when people patronise you . . . but it has led me to be more aware, to use this experience positively.
>
> (07M)

Important events in adulthood

For most students, men and women, social work was a career choice made in adulthood. Few of the students expected when they were children that they would grow up to become social workers – in fact, only three had heard of social work before they reached their late teens/early twenties. This meant that the majority of them came into social work after career and life experiences in other settings. It is here that gender differences emerge.

Women's experience prior to social work training is characterised by a narrow range of occupations, primarily centred on caring or service occupations, both paid and unpaid. Women had looked after children, and sometimes after parents and grandparents as well. Full-time carers had fitted in part-time work around their domestic responsibilities, often again in caring work, including childminding and foster care. Less frequently they had held other jobs such as taxi-driving, shop work or market research. Women without children had typically worked as office and administrative workers; as domestic bursars/wardens; and as residential or day-centre care workers (Figure 5.1).

Men's occupations prior to social work training were more varied than those of women, reflecting the wider opportunities available to men in all employment settings. Men had been everything from factory workers and engineers to lab technicians and farmers. None had been full-time carers at home, though eight had worked in paid caring jobs, as nurses, as residential workers and on one ocasion as a day-centre care assistant (Figure 5.1).

When men chose to change direction, this was often expressed in terms of the need for more autonomy, or for career development. They described feeling 'stuck' in their existing jobs (07M), or seeing social work as an 'interesting career with lots of jobs around' (08M). Some men who had worked in different caring settings in the past wanted 'more professional independence' (02M) in their work. One male student described how his attitude to hotel work changed as a result of being politicised:

> I thought this was terrible, this was not me at all. I really must change direction. My politics had changed completely, and I became more aware of the biases and prejudices that were going on in various people's lives that I had never come across before. So that's what motivated me initially to get into social

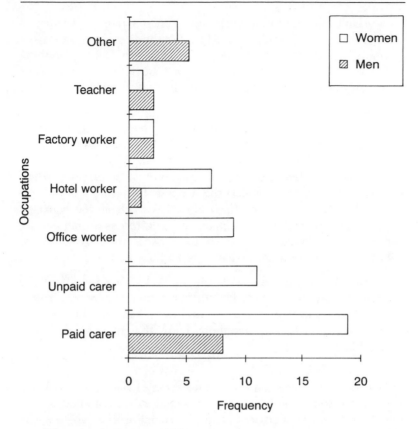

Figure 5.1 Previous occupations

work, into a more rewarding job, rather than being totally subservient to somebody over a reception desk. I was tired of having to paste on a smile in the mornings. I felt this was not real. Social work seems like a real job to me.

(25M)

The picture for women with children was very different. They tended to change direction after a period at home with children. The jobs which they had occupied before having children (in offices, shops or hospitals) no longer held attraction, and they looked for something new. This was most visible in situations where a marriage had broken up:

It wasn't really until the break-up of my marriage that I started to do things differently – I asked for the first time, what do I really need? It was quite clear that I was out doing everything for everybody else – there was no time to look at my own needs. So that's what made me go back into education.

(12F)

Sometimes the motivation for a change seems to be more pragmatic than anything else. Social work offered the opportunity of a career 'where I could earn a decent wage' (01F), and enjoy a measure of independence from the state or a former partner. It was also something which the women felt (through being a carer) that they knew something about. For others, the marriage itself, or the experience of bringing up children as a lone parent, was such that it led the women to reassess their lives, and to want to pass on to others what they had learned:

I think having to deal with the three kids by myself totally changed my views … being through what I've been through has changed my whole outlook on life … I had a pretty horrific marriage, and I'd like people to know that there's a life after all that.

(11F)

Two students (one male and one female) had quite personal reasons for switching to a career in social work. One had been a drug user, and wanted to become a social worker so that she could work with drug users (17F). The second, a born-again Christian, had experienced a calling from God (02M).

Results of the Occupational Decision Making questionnaire clarify the picture of difference and similarity between men and women in their career planning in adulthood. Both men and women consistently scored more highly on categories which related to the nature of the job itself (variety, creativity, responsibility) than on items such as pay and promotion in choosing social work as a career. The category which scored top for men and for women was personal fulfilment.

While all students tended to score job-related factors highly, there were gender differences related to specific questions. Women consistently rated supervision mechanisms as important in their career choice; some men did not. Men valued opportunities for leadership and promotion more highly than women.

Interestingly, there was little gender difference in questions which related to family-motivated factors. Women and men with young children gave equally high scores to flexible working hours, opportunities for part-time work and job share, and childcare availability. Younger students without dependants and those students whose children had grown up did not rate these as of any importance in their career choice.

(b) Perceptions of social work – social work as a women's profession

In spite of the fact that men are in a minority in social work (less than 30 per cent of this 1993–94 cohort of first-year students), neither men nor women tended to describe social work as a women's profession. Only three women and one man were willing to accept this characterisation. Behind this general statement, however, contradictory themes emerge. Women who rejected the idea that social work was a women's profession went on to say that women were 'better at it'. And many women (seven in total) volunteered that they believed clients prefer women social workers, whether in children and families' work, community care or social work with offenders.

This paradox demands further exploration. If women are 'better at it', and clients prefer women social workers, what do they mean by 'social work'? Do men and women see social work differently? I asked the students what they defined as the essential task of social work. Results varied, demonstrating no obvious gender differences. Most frequently students talked passionately about empowering people, about giving them choices, and about giving them back control of their lives. They also spoke about helping those in trouble, caring for others and respecting each person's humanity. Four women and three men bemoaned the current climate in social work, with its concentration on providing packages of care in a welfare bureaucracy. One man expressed this in matter-of-fact terms:

> I think the bottom line about social work is money, packages and competition. There is no way that it is going to be stopped unless there is a drastic change in policy, which is not going to happen.
>
> (25M)

A small number of students (men and women) were more concerned with changing the system than with caring for individuals within it:

> Social work isn't just about caring for people and not looking at the causes. I should be doing something to redress the balance, to fight, to go for the causes not the symptoms.
>
> (18M)

Although there were no gender differences in the ways in which students summed up the task of social work, there were profound differences in expectations about promotion. Ninety per cent of men in the individual interviews and all men in the group interviews stated that they expect to be promoted more quickly than women. While many said how unfair this was, and four said that they did not aspire to a promoted post, this perception was nevertheless considered to be factually correct: 'If you want to be a high-flier, it helps to be male' (16M). Women equally acknowledged that men's promotion prospects were better, and many were aware of the segregation which exists both within and across the profession of social work (Kravetz 1976; Howe 1986). But promotion prospects were not seen as the only area of advantage to men. Men also described other advantages based on gender:

> Because social work is not considered a male profession, it's as if there's not a protocol which is expected of you . . . you are open, freer as a man . . . there are not so many expectations of you.
>
> (04M)

Williams (1993), in a study of men in female-dominated occupations, takes up this point. She argues that for men in women's jobs, masculinity is a boon because 'qualities associated with men are more highly regarded than those associated with women, even in predominantly female jobs. . . . This fact reflects a widespread cultural prejudice that men are simply better than women' (Williams 1993: 3).

Research carried out twenty years ago into men in social work in the United States suggested that men move into administrative posts within social work in part as a strategy to cope with feelings of incongruity in a women's profession. Kadushin (1976) argued that men gravitate towards administrative and management positions as a way of spending more time with other men and in order to be more in touch with masculine modes of being. More recent research confirms this experience. Jacobs (1993) introduces the notion of 'revolving doors', examining how men are typically channelled and rechannelled out of female jobs and into better jobs that are more male-dominated. It is too early to see whether this prophecy will be fulfilled for this generation of student social workers. However, it is worth noting that men were as likely as women to express their work as 'nurturing' and seemed as comfortable as women with the caring aspects of social work.

Drawbacks of being a man in social work were identifed. Men described the pressure they experienced to adhere to traditional views of masculine behaviour. In residential care settings, they found that they were expected to be involved in physical restraint, where this was demanded. And they were disappointed that some of the more caring aspects of social work (particularly work with small children or with girls) were withheld from them. In social work training, they found themselves drawn into the role of spokespersons for the group, pushed forward by women students and receiving greater attention from staff because of their visibility. Whereas some men undoubtedly enjoyed this position, others did not.

In summary, social work, though largely staffed by women (especially at the level of hands-on caring), is not regarded as a 'women's profession' as such. This means that men in social work, while enjoying the advantages of being male in a non-traditional environment (better promotion and more autonomy), experience fewer difficulties than men in other women's settings such as nursing (Savage 1987; Williams 1989).

(c) Perceptions of self – men in social work

One explanation for men's ability to accept the caring bits of social work without experiencing status confusion or role strain might be that they are somehow different from other men. One male social work student expressed this very well:

> I sometimes look at myself, and this may sound sexist, but I always see myself as having picked up a lot of female characteristics. I have cared . . . I have a feeling for people.
>
> (19M)

A widespread phenomenon to emerge in interviews was that

men talked about feeling different in adolescence/young adulthood from their male peers. Half of the men whom I interviewed
said that they had never enjoyed conventional masculine activities
– 'football and pubbing' (18M) – and they felt more comfortable
in the company of women:

> Through my life most of my friends have been female. I play
> badminton, not football – a lot of girls here. And I like to talk
> about things. I do like to sit and chat and I enjoy social
> interaction. I probably prefer female company because I can
> be more *me* with girls or in a mixed group.
>
> (08M)

The high priority which many men in social work give to social
interaction is reflected in the results of the Occupational Decision
Making questionnaire. Here men scored social reasons for choosing social work as a career (that is, membership of a team,
friendship opportunities, leisure opportunities) as highly as
women. This may seem surprising, given the widely held psychological notion that women have greater commitment than men
to attachment and relationships (Gilligan 1982).

The Bem androgyny test (BSRI) offered an excellent opportunity to find out more about this identified feeling of being
different from other men. Here I found that men scored much
higher on the Femininity scale than men in Bem's original sample
of college students (Bem 1977). Whereas Bem's male students
were found to be feminine in less than 20 per cent of cases, male
social work students scored as feminine in 50 per cent of my
sample (see Table 5.2).

This result has been reproduced by other studies using the
BSRI which have examined men in non-traditional careers – that

Table 5.2 Results of male students on BSRI test as compared with
Bem's 1977 sample (percentages)

BSRI categories	Results from Scottish male social work student sample (%)	Bem's results from Stanford University student sample (%)
Masculine men	10	33
Feminine men	50	17
Androgynous men	30	25
Undifferentiated men	10	25

is, careers which have less than 30 per cent of same-sex workers. Chusmir's summary of research findings shows that men who choose female-dominated occupations are likely to possess many of the same traits and characteristics often attributed to women in the same jobs (Chusmir 1990). Studies by Russell (1983) and Rosenwasser and Patterson (1984–85) found that men who have assumed the role of househusband are more likely to be androgynous than men in general. Pontin's study of male and female nurses draws similar conclusions (Pontin 1988). More recently, Galbraith (1992) has discovered that men in elementary education tend to be classified less often as masculine and more often as feminine than their male peers in both nursing and engineering.

So where does this lead us? Is the hypothesis that men in the caring professions are different from other men proved? I would doubt it. What we can be sure about is that the men *see themselves* as different from other men. They have embraced characteristics commonly held to be feminine, and are not afraid to call them their own. There is a correspondence with the interview findings and with analysis of the results of the BSRI and the Occupational Decision Making questionnaire. In all these arenas, the male students illustrate attitudes and beliefs about themselves which have routinely been associated with female attributes, including a concern for friendship, intimacy and responsibility. At the same time, men have not given up their male qualities – hence their greater interest in promotion, and their relatively high androgynous scores.

Implications for social work

To return to my initial question, 'Why do men care?', my answer is unequivocal. My research study has shown that although men and women may share similar childhood experiences which lead them to have an interest in and a concern for helping others, the gendered nature of society means that beyond this common starting point there are profound gender differences for men and women in social work. Men who choose to become social workers do so in the knowledge that they are different – that they have qualities which are not stereotypically held to be male. This realisation gives them the possibility of greater differentiation and greater scope in their work with clients and colleagues. Men also enter social work with the confidence that their promotion prospects (should they choose to take advantage of them) are higher than those of women.

Women, on the other hand, in becoming social workers are pursuing a career which draws on characteristics which are widely held to be feminine. One woman student put this simply: 'by taking on the caring role, I'm reinforcing the whole idea of women and caring' (17F). And women know that their promotion prospects are lower than those of men (Crompton and Sanderson 1990), even though many women respondents said that they would like a senior or management post in the future.

There are a number of challenges leading on from this for social work education and for social work as a whole. First, I believe that we should welcome men who are willing to criticise conventional, 'macho' models of masculine behaviour, and who are prepared to express an alternative, more 'feminine' version of masculinity. Women and men have a lot to gain from the process of critically examining both masculine and feminine categories and stereotypes. But two important qualifications must be made here. First, we should not fall into the trap of congratulating men for being caring men, valuing them for qualities which we routinely expect of women. And second, any exploration of gender conditioning must be underpinned by a political awareness of the sexist and patriarchal nature of British society. Men's experience of gender oppression can never be equated with that of women, although connections can indeed be made in terms of oppression based on sexual orientation, class, race and disability (Ramazanoğlu 1989).

Another area which demands urgent attention is the reappraisal of the 'feminine' side of social work. Social work practice is rapidly becoming more technical, more bureaucratic, more 'masculine' in style, whether carried out by men or by women, and my research has shown that it is the personal, caring, 'feminine' aspects of social work which both women and men social work students see as most worthwhile. This is not, of course, to suggest that only men feel comfortable with the notion of contracts and competencies and care-plans. But it is to argue that the pressure on outcomes and male-dominated strategic language can lose sight of the importance of feelings and values, of self-insight and inter-personal relationships in social work practice.

A third theme which has emerged in my research is the very different impact on men and women of their own caring responsibilities before and during social work training. Women are more likely to enter social work training with a background in caring for others. Once on the course, they are more likely to be principal carers, and are often lone parents looking after children. If social work management is concerned to get the best candidates for its senior posts, and if social work as a profession is genuinely committed to equal opportunities, then we must find ways of valuing and supporting women's caring in the family, and of understanding the political significance of personal caring. This will inevitably mean developing more flexible institutional arrangements for patterns of work and for the organisation of practice placements. It will also require a greater recognition of the importance of caring at the point of selection to social work training. Social work and educational institutions are unlikely to make the necessary changes without a struggle. This is the challenge for those of us who are feminists working in social work.

APPENDIX

(a) Occupational Decision-Making Questionnaire

Instructions: Indicate on a scale of 1 to 7 how important each of the following factors is in your decision to become a professional social worker. A 1 means the item is not at all important, and a 7 means that it is extremely important to you.

1 income
2 independence/autonomy
3 variety
4 membership of a team
5 interesting work
6 supervision mechanisms
7 socially useful work
8 friendship opportunities
9 responsibility
10 creativity

11 status/prestige
12 job security
13 childcare availability
14 leadership opportunities
15 leisure opportunities
16 flexible working hours
17 opportunities for part-time/ job-share
18 promotion opportunities
19 pension fund
20 personal fulfilment

Source: Adapted from Boreham and Arthur 1993

(b) Bem Sex Role Inventory

Instructions: Indicate on a scale of 1 to 7 how well each of the following characteristics describes you. A 1 means the item is never or almost never true, and a 7 means that it is always or almost always true (Bem 1974).

1 self-reliant	23 sympathetic	41 warm
2 yielding	24 jealous	42 solemn
3 helpful	25 has leadership abilities	43 willing to take a stand
4 defends own beliefs	26 sensitive to needs of others	44 tender
5 cheerful		45 friendly
6 moody	27 truthful	46 aggressive
7 independent	28 willing to take risks	47 gullible
8 shy		48 inefficient
9 conscientious	29 understanding	49 acts as a leader
10 athletic	30 secretive	50 childlike
11 affectionate	31 makes decisions easily	51 adaptable
12 theatrical		52 individualistic
13 assertive	32 compassionate	53 does not use harsh language
14 flatterable	33 sincere	
15 happy	34 self-sufficient	54 unsystematic
16 strong personality	35 eager to soothe hurt feelings	55 competitive
17 loyal		56 loves children
18 unpredictable	36 conceited	57 tactful
19 forceful	37 dominant	58 ambitious
20 feminine	38 soft spoken	59 gentle
21 reliable	39 likeable	60 conventional
22 analytical	40 masculine	

Chapter 6

Interviewing violent men
Challenge or compromise?

Kate Cavanagh and Ruth Lewis[1]

CONTEXTUALISING OUR EXPERIENCE

For the last three years we have been talking to violent men. All 122 of them have been through the court system for an offence involving violence against their female partner.[2] Some have been fined, some admonished; others have been placed on probation or placed on a men's programme as a special condition of their probation order. A few have been imprisoned. These men have been abusing their partners physically, emotionally and sexually, some for years. We talked to them about their lives, thoughts and feelings about their behaviour and their relationships with the women they have been abusing. We spent over 300 hours listening to men excuse, deny, minimise and blame. Some have cried, some have raged, some have laughed, some have flirted, some have challenged. Some have sought to humour us, to enlist our sympathy, to control us, to outsmart us, to convince us.

This work has inevitably altered our way of seeing the world, particularly our way of seeing men. As feminists, we were acutely aware of the contentious nature of the task we undertook: in many ways feminists have been reluctant to work with and conduct research on men. This is understandable. Our priority should always be with women. However, the core of women's oppression cannot be understood and changed by focusing on women alone, and we believe that feminists must include direct work with men as part of their agenda for change.

This chapter begins by exploring the issues which we confronted when we worked on a research project whose wider remit was to undertake a longitudinal and comparative evaluation of two men's programmes for perpetrators of domestic violence.

This evaluation was based on interviews with men and women, and two follow-up postal questionnaires. We will not address the specific questions which the evaluation was designed to explore. What we will do in this chapter is discuss our experiences as feminist researchers working with men. What have we learned about men that might be useful for other women, for other feminists? What new ideas have occurred to us in the course of doing this work? We consider some of the dilemmas we struggled with as we attempted to integrate 'thinking' feminist research with 'doing' feminist research. Finally, we consider the impact that talking to violent men had on us personally.

DOMESTIC VIOLENCE AND MEN'S PROGRAMMES – SETTING THE SCENE

The research and literature in the area of woman abuse has significantly increased in the last twenty years, a development substantially influenced by the women's movement and its many activists. They have raised public awareness of the numerous ways in which men control, dominate and intimidate their partners. The debates within this field have been many but none has been more contentious than the issue of work with perpetrators (Dobash and Dobash 1992; Hague and Malos 1993). Until very recently, perpetrators have remained largely invisible to all – including the criminal justice system. The concern for the safety of abused women and the welfare of their children has rightly been given priority in responses to domestic violence. Unquestionably, there is no substitute for providing safety, accommodation and assistance for abused women. However, if the abuser is not to repeat his violence, then attention must also be turned to how his violence might be stopped. By failing to focus on the *perpetrators* of violence the source of the problem is left unaddressed and the problem is reproduced, with tragic consequences.

Changes in some men's violent behaviour have undoubtedly occurred as a consequence of women's resistance and challenge. In North America attempts to work directly with the perpetrators of domestic violence began over a decade ago. There are now hundreds of men's programmes (Eisikovits and Edleson 1989; Burns *et al.* 1991). However, some feminists have viewed such developments with scepticism: will men's programmes eventually overshadow services for women? Will there be competition for resources? In North America, developments in services for men often coexist uncomfortably with services for women (Adams 1988; Hart 1988). In Britain, the discourse around men's programmes has begun and the debate is no less heated within the feminist community. As Hague and Malos point out, 'There is a lot of doubt in the refuge movement as to whether men's programmes, especially the therapeutic ones, can work' (Hague and Malos 1993: 193).

The critical issue to be considered when thinking about programmes for perpetrators is change. Do these programmes work? Are men less violent, abusive and intimidating as a consequence of participating in these programmes? Such questions have been unanswered because evaluations of the effectiveness of programmes have been minimal and, of the few which have been conducted, most have been fraught with severe design and methodological problems (Dobash, Dobash, Cavanagh and Lewis 1995a). There is general agreement that thorough evaluations of the effectiveness of the programmes are vital, and many activists, whilst being broadly supportive of programmes, await the results of evaluations.

OUR EVALUATION

It was within this contentious political climate that the evaluation project we were involved in began. The men's programmes we evaluated were the first of their kind in Europe and their growth coincided with a move within Scottish social work towards raising the priority of work with offenders.[3] Social work with offenders including men's programmes is now receiving considerable funding and attention.

Scotland saw the development of the first men's programmes in the United Kingdom. The CHANGE[4] Programme and the Lothian Domestic Violence Probation Programme began in 1990 and 1991 respectively. These new initiatives were born only after considerable negotiations with Scottish Women's Aid. Both programmes are pro-feminist and re-educational. They are also multi-agency initiatives; each operates collaboratively with police, health, social work and criminal justice agencies as well as local Women's Aid groups. From the beginning, all those involved in establishing the programmes were united in requiring that these programmes be evaluated. After several unsuccessful applications, funding was eventually secured and our project instigated.[5] There were five of us in the research team: the Principal Investigators, Russell and Rebecca Dobash, were based in Cardiff; ourselves, the research associates who along with our project administrator, Pat Young, were based in Scotland. In its broadest sense our evaluation was designed to assess and compare the impact of a range of criminal justice sanctions on men's violent behaviour. The principal research question was, 'Do the new innovative programmes lead to changes in men's violent and abusive behaviour?' The research was also designed to explore why men change and to examine the factors associated with this.

FEMINIST RESEARCH

We came to this research as feminists and therefore we considered that we were 'doing feminist research'. Feminist ideas and understanding informed the project design and methodology (Dobash and Dobash 1979, 1983, 1988). However, from the beginning, our involvement in this project was not without problems. Why was researching men so problematic? Before answering this question it is necessary briefly to contextualise our discussion in terms of the current feminist epistemological and methodological debates.

Over the last twenty years feminists have constructed a powerful critique of social science knowledge (Dobash and Dobash 1979, 1983, 1988; Stanley and Wise 1983; Rose 1986; Harding 1987; Reinharz 1992). Feminist enquiry has energised and problematized debates about 'knowledge' and 'truth' and has made such enquiry more widely accessible to influences outside academia. By emphasising the importance of experience in developing theory, questions of 'knowledge' became the legitimate property of all women whose explication of their own experiences laid a foundation for much of the new feminist scholarship.

In the last decade, distinct criticisms of the traditional 'scientific method', such as the exclusion of women and women's experiences and an over-reliance on quantitative methods, have been raised by feminist researchers (Fonow and Cook 1992; Reinharz 1992; Stanley and Wise 1993). Postmodernist ideas emphasising notions of difference and diversity have also been extremely influential in feminist theory (Weedon 1987; Hekman 1990;

Lather 1991). Acknowledgement of the diversity of women and recognition of the difficulties produced by seeking to verify a common theory of oppression have fuelled much recent feminist thinking (Ramazanoğlu 1989; Grant 1993). While the acceptability of difference is now more fully integrated into current feminist thought, some suggest that the focus on difference and diversity has masked 'the importance of power differentials and relations' (Gordon 1991: 92). Many researchers and activists are concerned that the fragmented nature of the feminist academic discourse has created a growing schism between theoretical feminism and political activism (Kelly et al. 1994). Ramazanoğlu asserts that, 'we cannot afford to wholly abandon a sense of sisterhood. Without it there can be no basis for a feminist politics' (1989: 175).

As researchers struggling to comprehend the complex theoretical debates around epistemological difference, in common with other feminist researchers, we found ourselves dejected by the 'pessimism of theory' (Kelly et al. 1994: 26). Though intellectually very challenging, such debates seemed surreal when juxtaposed alongside the continuing abusive and oppressive reality of many women's lives. Thus, whilst it was important that we explore the feminist epistemological literature in order to locate a framework to contextualise our own fieldwork, predictably more questions were raised than answers provided. Nevertheless, these debates formed the backdrop to our work as feminist researchers.

Two other developments were significant for us. The first concerned the area of 'men and masculinity'. The study of men and masculinity has been significantly influenced by feminism. Whereas some men have supported feminist ideas and criticisms and have sought to examine and change the nature of oppressive masculine practices (Connell 1987; Hearn 1987; Brittan 1989), others have responded more defensively (Hodson 1984; Ford 1985; Walczak 1988). However, it has been suggested that the reponse of many men 'has been one of a diffuse if rarely articulated opposition' (Morgan 1992: 10). Generally, women have been sceptical of the motivation underlying the growth of the 'men's movement' (Friedman and Sarah 1982). The more recent emergence of an anti-feminist literature (Bly 1991; Lyndon 1992) has concerned many feminists (Hagan 1992), and more are entering the debate about the nature of men and masculinity (Segal 1990a; Phillips 1993).

The second development relates to domestic violence and is integrally related to the previous point. Some men's programmes were initially established by men loosely affiliated to the men's movement (Hart 1988; Dobash and Dobash 1992). Women's involvement in these programmes has been extremely varied; some feminists were influential in establishing pro-feminist-based programmes many of which were staffed by men and women, whilst other programmes were staffed exclusively by men. The concerns from feminists (Hart 1988) are that the absence of women from these programmes may result in collusion between counsellors and perpetrators. It is extremely important that the experiences of women who have been abused inform not only programmes but also any research into the evaluation of the effectiveness of these programmes.

Refocusing our 'feminist lens'

There is no one particular model or definition of feminist research, but most feminists would agree that what is fundamental is theoretical location (Maynard 1994). We believed that what made our work feminist was the 'feminist lens' (Grant 1993: 103) through which we tried to make sense of men's worlds. However, we felt it was important to explore those themes appearing in the literature which were particularly relevant to our work with men. One of the questions we found ourselves continually asking was, 'Does researching men change the essence of these themes and if so, what implications does this have for developing feminist research theory and practice for the future?'

Researching men

Understanding and articulating the ways in which women are oppressed by men has constituted the backbone of feminist research. However, just as this articulation inevitably provokes questions about the nature and reality of women's lives it also leads us to examine the nature of men's lives. Nevertheless, researching men's lives is 'a relatively underdeveloped aspect of feminist research' (Maynard 1994: 15) though more feminists are now acknowledging the need to develop new insights into men's worlds (Scully 1990; Stanko 1994).

Method

Qualitative methods have come to be seen as synonymous with feminist research because they offer the potential to explore the meanings of experience. One question from this debate was important for our work. How willing would violent men be to explore their violence in depth? As a team, we were convinced of the value of using both quantitative and qualitative approaches (Dobash and Dobash 1981; Dobash *et al.* 1995b). We also knew from activists and practitioners (Pence and Paymar 1990; personal communications with activists) that men would be reluctant to discuss their violence in depth and therefore we had to devise a data-gathering instrument which took account of these considerations. We discuss the interview schedule in more detail later.

Relationships

Many feminists (Kelly 1988; Oakley 1981) have been critical of the ways in which much traditional sociological research has involved hierarchical power relationships and an objectification and exploitation of the respondent. Some have highlighted the need not only to acknowledge and minimise power differentials but also to democratise the research process.[6] Although we were committed to the idea of minimising power differentials with women, this stance seemed inappropriate with men. Maintaining power and control seemed to be important features of our work with these men.

Action research and the role of the researcher

Fundamental to much feminist research is the concept of action; a belief that the recommendations which follow the research should lead to change which will positively affect women's lives (Dobash and Dobash 1981). In our study, effecting long-term change was an important objective. However, short-term change was also a consideration. Should we attempt, for example, to raise men's awareness of how their behaviour and attitudes might have impacted on the women they had abused? We had to consider how compromised we would feel if, in the course of interviewing men, we failed to challenge responses which reflected patriarchal ideas and attitudes. However, we had to balance this against the need to collect valid research data.

As a research team, reflecting on all of these themes made us think more critically about methods, about our role as interviewers and about the ways in which these ideas might help us construct a methodological framework which we could use in our interviews with violent men.

OUR WORK WITH MEN

The project began in June 1991 and ended in June 1994.[7] During that time we interviewed 122 men and 146 women. The interviews with the women were a critical part of the evaluation. Much of the literature on men's programmes in North America indicates that many men will minimise their abuse (Adams 1988; Sinclair 1989). Therefore any information we obtained from men had to be compared to accounts of abuse obtained from their partner.

We accessed cases involving domestic violence through the court records.[8] Men and women were initially contacted by post and asked if they would be willing to participate. Relatively few responded immediately, and we subsequently visited each individual at home seeking their cooperation.

We conducted almost all the interviews individually and all but a few were carried out in the homes of the participants. We always sought to interview men and women separately when partners were not at home. In all situations we were alert to the woman's sense of safety and security. If a woman indicated that she felt an interview would threaten her safety or security, we withdrew. Where women expressed any reservations about their partners being interviewed, we would not proceed any further.

The majority of the men were young adults between the ages of twenty and thirty-five, white, working class and often unemployed. Most were fathers and were usually still living with their partner. The interviews with men were lengthy, typically lasting about two hours and all respondents were advised that the interviews would cover sensitive areas of their lives. All the interviews were tape-recorded.

Our interview schedule was over fifty pages long and comprised of a range of structured and semi-structured questions about many aspects of the man's life. For example, we asked men about their backgrounds, their social networks, their relationships

with their partner, their attitudes towards women, their involvement in family life, the nature and frequency of their violent
and controlling behaviour towards their partner, attribution of
responsibility associated with conflict, their prior attempts to stop
or reduce their abusive behaviour and the response of others to
the abuse and the effect of this on their future behaviour.

Interviewing violent men: challenge and critical engagement

As we struggled to develop ideas which would inform our
research practice, the concept of challenge became a particularly
important theme for us. We believed that challenge was an essential part of our work with violent men, and we concluded that it
was important for us to develop methods which focused upon
challenge within the interviewer–respondent relationship.[9] We
looked at how other researchers doing similar work had
approached this issue. Diane Scully (1990), who interviewed convicted rapists, emphasised the difficulties she experienced in
developing the interviewer–respondent relationship. She
described herself as 'an interested, supportive, non-judgmental
outsider' who treated the men as 'experts' (1990: 17). Though
she found it extremely difficult to remain neutral, she felt that to
be otherwise might compromise her ultimate goal of acquiring
reliable data.

The aim of another pro-feminist writer who interviewed domestic violence perpetrators was 'to effect a narrative rather than
continually challenge the men' (Ptacek 1988: 137). Although he
believed confrontation could be an effective strategy in bringing
about change, he felt that as an interviewing style it would be
likely to produce superficial, defensive and dishonest responses.
He chose to challenge after the interview when he became the
'confrontative counsellor' (Ptacek 1988: 138), a position he felt it
was safe to adopt after the collection of reliable data. This 'impar-
tial' approach also posed questions for us. For example, would it
be possible for us to listen to men's accounts of their violence
towards their partners and remain 'neutral'? Would we not be
reinforcing men's justifications of their violence if we accepted
their explanations unquestioningly? The very important difference between Ptacek's approach and our own is epitomised in
his comment, 'We pretty much looked at each other straight

in the eye in a very clear expression of connection. We clearly trusted each other' (Ptacek 1988: 140).

Aware that society does little to condemn men's violence towards women, we felt that it would be unjustifiable to take such a 'hands-off' approach. We knew that to seek to 'change' our respondents was competely unrealistic; this was not our objective as researchers. However, as we did not permit sexist remarks to go unchallenged in other areas of our lives, why should we in our role as researchers? The practice literature on violent men (Adams 1988; Pence and Paymar 1990) suggests that men are extremely reluctant to explore their behaviour and to move beyond superficial responses. We wished to enrich our understanding of men's perceptions of their own behaviour and attitudes. Challenge was then important not only on a political and ethical basis, but also as a methodological technique; potentially it could provide us with more fulsome data. We viewed it as a means of penetrating beyond the denying, minimising and blaming behaviour that men are accustomed to displaying. Challenge might encourage a man to justify a statement and then consider the assumptions underpinning that statement. Contrary to some opinions that challenge 'contaminates data' (Ptacek 1988: 138), we believed that men who were not questioned critically are in fact more likely to say what they think the interviewer wants to hear. Reinharz states that when feminists 'study up' (1992: 42), they are likely to demand less. We wanted to demand *more*. Rather than being passive listeners and recorders of information, we wished to integrate our feminist perspective into the interview process; to construct a form of enquiry which enabled us to question men about their violence without alienating them. We felt we were charting new territory, by attempting to extend the boundaries of feminist research with men. Whilst excited by this prospect, we were also apprehensive.

Preparation

Preparation was an essential aspect of the interviewing. The interviews were lengthy and emotionally and physically draining. We had to prepare ouselves psychologically for these encounters with men. This became particularly difficult if we had interviewed a man's partner first and had learned the full extent of his abusive behaviour. Women's accounts were often extremely detailed and harrowing, and it was at times difficult to conceal our disbelief at the minimal accounts given by their partners. The accounts of men and women were often so contradictory that we wondered how it was possible that these two people could inhabit the same relationship.

We wanted to establish an interview role which was both effective and comfortable and this also affected ideas about how we would physically appear to men. We pondered together on the most appropriate dress for these interviews, opting for trousers rather than skirts, avoiding jewellery or make-up. We struggled with the desire to avoid any suggestion of flippancy or sexual attractiveness while also wanting to challenge men's stereotypical views of women.

We were aware that interacting with violent men and asking them to expose the full extent of their abuse could be risky. At the beginning of the project, whilst we were developing the questionnaire, we rarely discussed the possibility of risk. Looking back, we both felt that we should be able to 'handle ourselves'. We assumed that men who abuse their partners are rarely abusive to others except perhaps their children. However, as we ploughed through three years of sheriff court records, we soon found that some men who abuse their partners *can* be violent to others. And with this knowledge now, we might have reconsidered the rather casual view we had about risk.

We spent endless hours, day and night, walking the streets seeking to enlist our respondents. The 'doorstep' sell became a routine research practice. We never knew what kind of response we would meet once the door was opened. We therefore had to be continually prepared and alert. However, although we were subjected to a certain amount of verbal abuse from men, only very occasionally did we ever feel at any physical risk. Sometimes we were alerted to information, for example, from the court record or one of the programme coordinators, which indicated that interviewing this man might be particularly risky. On these rare occasions we either decided not to interview or we conducted the interview together.

The role which we set out to adopt in interviews presented us with a constant dilemma. Were we sufficiently challenging? Did men ever think we agreed with their explanations, did they tell us what they thought we wanted to hear? Did we ever lose men's co-operation because we were too challenging? In retrospect we realise that it was an area in which we had to compromise in several ways.

Initially, the research team felt strongly that our approach to men who had been violent had to be open and honest. We could not 'trick' them into talking to us. From the outset, we wanted men to be aware that we were there to talk about their abusive behaviour. So, in our introductory letters inviting them to participate in the research, we referred to their violent behaviour towards their partner and the subsequent court case. We felt it was important that they were fully aware of the purpose of the interview. We could have been less direct; we could have used numerous euphemisms for violence, referring to an 'incident' or an 'event' or the 'offence', but we felt that such an approach could lead to misunderstanding. We could potentially be confronted by an angry man who may have completely misunderstood the purpose of the interview. A few men responded angrily to our letter, some protesting that they had not been violent to their partners, that they had 'just' been sentenced for breach of the peace, that it was 'all a mistake'. Quickly we rephrased the letter. This early experience jolted us from our ideological pedestal. We realised that if we were to get men to talk to us, we had to seek to engage with them positively. This, of course, had its problems.

Critical engagement

All interviewers in the social sciences recognise the importance of building rapport. Without this, the possibility of acquiring 'valid' data is diminished. Violent men often present to others as plausible, blameless individuals. Many are extremely well guarded and defended (Adams 1988; Pence and Paymar 1990). We wanted to penetrate this façade, to facilitate open discussion. We also anticipated much resistance. Developing rapport was therefore essential for our work. Rapport and challenge are intimately yet incongruously linked; each threatens to endanger the other. If we challenged without establishing rapport, the man might become angry or uncooperative. Challenge and rapport were therefore key themes and had to be constantly balanced. However, developing challenge whilst effecting and maintaining rapport are not uncontradictory objectives and, whilst rapport was an essential component of our interviews, it was also a problematic concept. If we accept that rapport often depends on empathy, how questionable or possible is it for feminists to empathise, to create a supportive atmosphere, to communicate an understanding and acceptance of a man who uses violence against his partner? The concept of 'engagement' seemed more appropriate than rapport. Engaging suggested connection without empathy or acceptance, and, when qualified by 'critical', it became a working construct which we felt adequately communicated the key elements of our methods. Thus challenge and critical engagement became constant features throughout the planning and conducting of interviews.

Engaging with men was probably less onerous than we had expected. The ability to engage with our male respondents raises the issue of the gender of the interviewer. We felt that engagement was less of a problem because we were women; men are unaccustomed to talking about intimate, personal aspects of their lives and when they venture to do so, it is usually with mothers, partners, sisters, daughters, social workers – women.

Some men did, in fact, present as extremely plausible, convincing and charming. We liked many of them. In talking to some of them, we were able to appreciate and understand the strong connections that some women have to their partners. Many were relatively easy to engage, particularly at the start of the interview where we had deliberately placed less emotionally charged questions. With these men, it was more difficult to indicate our intention that the rest of the interview might not be so easy-going; some men were more difficult to challenge and became more defensive to our questions. Conversely, those men who were less concerned with presenting themselves as charming were sometimes more difficult to engage but were perhaps easier to challenge as they appeared to have fewer defences.

A key concern was that we might sympathise too much with the men and thereby lose the 'critical' part of engagement. An important part of doing any work with abusive men is resisting the invitation to collude with them. Such men often become accomplished manipulators; interviewers and practitioners need to be prepared to recognise and resist this.[10] The line between colluding and empathising is a fine one. For example, when men talked about aspects of their lives which were removed from their abusive behaviour – police harassment because of their involvement with illegal drugs, the misery of long-term unemployment, the desperate state of their council accommodation, poor medical treatment of their children – it is difficult and, indeed, undesirable to ignore the very real impact of these experiences. However, whilst we sympathised with men regarding such aspects of their lives we would question their use of such experiences to *justify* their violence. Some men grasped this distinction and this helped to establish a good working relationship. Indeed, the ability to sympathise with men regarding such experiences improved rapport, enabled challenge and so helped develop critical engagement.

The interviews with women were essential in that they helped us maintain our critical edge with men. Without the imput of the women, we could have been drawn into compromising or colluding with men. Once more, the necessity for this work to be informed by women's experiences was highlighted.

Some techniques which researchers use for building rapport, we found, were not appropriate when engaging with violent men. For example, we were extremely careful about the use of humour. Men often used humour to minimise the seriousness of their behaviour. A common excuse cited was that women 'bruise easily'. This was often followed by a laugh. Whilst mirroring this response might build rapport by easing tension and thereby facilitate fuller disclosure, men could just as easily interpret such a response as an affirmation of their own view. On such occasions our strategy was not to reciprocate with humour but to ask questions which explored this answer in more depth. This does not mean that we presented as intense, humourless interviewers. Humour was used to engage men and ease the tension which talking about something like personal violence inevitably produces but it was not used in response to the humour men used to minimise their behaviour. The use of irony was problematic for similar reasons.

Techniques of challenge

The apprehension we experienced in developing our roles as challenging interviewers was paralleled by the uneasiness of our male respondents in their role. Most men were clearly uncomfortable when talking in detail about an aspect of their behaviour of which they were ashamed. Despite their wide range of intricate excuses and denials, most of the men *did* feel shame, though their ability and willingness to express this shame varied. Some felt uneasy when they realised that the excuses and denials usually proferred to partners, family members, criminal justice personnel, doctors and social workers would not be so easily accepted in the unique context of a research interview.

We predicted that their discomfort and reluctance would limit their responses to monosyllabic answers. For many men, being expected to articulate emotions, ideas and behaviours which they thought they were unaware or unsure of or unable to name is, in itself, a challenge. Many women stated that their men were 'deep'. This generally meant that the men rarely talked about their emotions. We are not arguing that our male respondents were any different from most men in this respect. Simply, we recognised that talking about this sensitive subject would be extremely difficult for these men. In order to gather more meaningful data than a series of 'yes–no–depends' responses we had to devise techniques which would encourage them to express themselves fully.

To clarify what we understand by challenge, we place challenge somewhere between probing and confrontation. It is a technique which can make use of standard probing questions but avoids outright confrontation. Challenge can be used to explore sensitive issues with reluctant respondents. It can be a technique for exploring and developing answers beyond the 'yes–no–depends' responses. We used several techniques to effect challenge.

Challenges could be subtle. For example, when a man makes a statement that he thinks is a 'taken-for-granted' fact, it could be a simple 'What makes you say that?' Alternatively, it could be a rephrasing of his statement as a question, 'So *you* think that . . .', emphasising that it is *his* opinion rather than a 'fact':

I: Who do you think was responsible for the violence that time?

R: Eh, I'd say both of us, well if she'd left us alane that night nothing would have happened, if she'd let us come in, put the stuff away, go tae ma bed [but] then she started arguing 'where have you been?' and that, an' ah just exploded.

I: So you 'just exploded'?

R: I think that was it, yeh, it just blew up fae there. I wisnae havin her comin' in and givin' me hassle.

Challenge can also involve referring to some earlier comment and asking him to rethink it in the light of later comments:

> *I:* Can I ask you about something you told me earlier on? You said that amongst working class people it's not acceptable to hit women yet you've hit a woman, your wife. How do you explain that?
>
> *R:* I've never hit another woman. If it's yer wife it's OK, it's different if it's yer wife. But ye never hit a woman like in the street or in a pub.

Another technique can be asking a man to consider how a certain type of behaviour affects his partner:

> *I:* How did you feel after that [violent] incident?
>
> *R:* Just felt relieved.
>
> *I:* Relieved after you'd done that? (*Smashed house up, threatened friends, threw TV out of window, threatened to do same to partner.*)
>
> *R:* Well I didn't hit her, you know what I mean.
>
> *I:* You threatened her though.
>
> *R:* Aye, but I didn't raise my hands to her.
>
> *I:* But you threatened her. You probably frightened her.
>
> *R:* Aye, I got her feared.... I was a bit ashamed of myself when I look back on it.

A further approach is to question a man's logic:

> *I:* Can you remember the very first time [you hit ——]?
>
> *R:* Em, I was walking doon the stairs one day after I'd been drinking.
>
> *I:* Hmm.
>
> *R:* I was pure steaming and she laughed at us and I went to the knives and that.
>
> *I:* You went for?
>
> *R:* The knives and chased her oot the hoose. When I think about the knife, I think that was just to gie' her a fright you know, I wouldnae use it.
>
> *I:* Do you think she knew that?
>
> *R:* Aye, cause ... she said, 'gi' me that', you know, took it off us.
>
> *I:* So even though you were steaming and you often black out, you can still be sure you'd never use a knife?
>
> *R:* No, I couldnae be sure I wouldnae use it.
>
> *I:* So surely *she* can't be sure you're not going to use it?
>
> *R:* True, aye.

Some men found it difficult to answer questions or were firmly resistant to expanding on their responses. In these cases, probing could work to provide us with a more detailed picture of a man's opinions and attitudes, enabling us to gather fuller data about the justifications for his behaviour. These justifications provided us with much insight into these men's understanding of the world:

I: Why do you hit her?
R: Just to get her to do what I think is right.
I: So to get her to do what you want.
R: Aye.
I: And why should you want her to do that?
R: Because she's ma wife.
I: Does that give you the right to expect her to do your bidding?
R: In my book, yes.

As we became more experienced in using and developing the technique of challenge, we came to appreciate the cumulative impact this seemed to have over the course of the interview; some men came to recognise the exploratory thread running throughout the interviews: one man even pre-empted the interviewer's question by asking *himself,* 'I know, "what makes you say that?" ' The importance of using challenge lies in assisting men to move beyond their superficial responses and encouraging them to explore the meaning of their behaviour and the attitudes and beliefs underpinning them. While individual challenges might not appear particularly dynamic, the probing context within which they are used can make an important contribution to the overall effect.

Maximising men's responses

Challenge was a very useful technique for uncovering men's minimisation of their behaviour. However, it was very important that we establish the nature and extent of men's violence towards their partners in order to assess and uncover the extent to which change had occurred. This required that we talk to men in some depth about the details of the acts of violence, and this proved to be one of the areas where men exploited their ability to minimise to the fullest degree.[11] In anticipation of this, the research team devised 'incidence cards'. On one card was a list of various types of violence and on a separate card a list of types of injuries. Each act of violence (twenty-six separate acts listed) and type of injury (twenty-six types of injury listed) was placed alongside a letter. Below are extracts from the cards.

Violence Assessment Index

A   Restrain her from moving or leaving the room
M   Punch or kick the walls or furniture
P   Force her to have sex or some kind of sexual activity

Injury Assessment Index

A   Cut/s on her face
E   Broken arm or leg
S   Split lip

Men were given the card, we read out the letter and they were asked to tell us, by answering 'yes or no' if they had committed the act or if their partner had sustained the injury. In practice, we found that these cards facilitated the collection of much more detailed information from the men. Before introducing the cards, we used an open-ended question to ask them to describe a violent incident; the typical response was a scant, minimal version of events:

> *I*:   Can you remember what happened the last time that you assaulted her?
> *R*:   Just hit her – there had been an argument.
> *I*:   Can you remember what happened?
> *R*:   Just started to argue and I just lashed out. I think I picked something up and hit her.
> *I*:   Can you remember anything else?
> *R*:   The polis came and took me away.

However, by using the cards, the man in the example above was able to 'remember' his violent actions in greater detail. He had restrained his partner, punched her in the face, slapped, pushed and grabbed her, threatened and hit her with a metal bar and with his fist, thrown things at her, shouted, screamed, sworn at her, called her names, and threatened to kill her. Her injuries included a cut and bleeding face, bruised body and face, nausea and unconsciousness.

Importantly, we were able to elicit this information without forcing the men to 'name' their behaviour and without confrontation. We expected that men would be extremely reluctant to describe their abusive behaviours towards their partner. We had to find a means of talking about violent behaviour without relying constantly on euphemisms – for example 'incident' or 'occasion' for 'violent event'. This often occurred at the beginning of an interview, then, depending on the degree of engagement, we would bring more direct language into the questioning. Non-confrontational, yet challenging devices such as these can provide feminist researchers and practitioners with an important repertoire of techniques with which to approach work with (violent) men.

Challenge and confrontation

Challenge should not be confused with confrontation. Where challenge can encourage a man to explore his attitudes, confrontation can be risky both for the interviewer and the man's partner especially if the man feels 'badgered' or 'provoked'. Confrontation can also reinforce sexist attitudes and we were extremely careful not to confront men. We did not rely on continuous probing which could lead to confrontation. In fact, we used the interview schedule to do some of this challenging for us. The research team designed the interview schedule to question men's minimisation and denial of their violence as much as possible and to do so with minimal reliance on confrontation. The selection, phrasing and ordering of questions were carefully considered. Questions were simple and direct and the range of issues covered thoughtfully planned, so that the sensitive issues were interspersed with the more mundane to reduce the potential for the build-up of tension and emotion. Challenges were built into the questionnaire and focused on issues such as the impact of the man's behaviour on others. The following questions were integrated into the questionnaire and were asked of all men:

Q4   When you hit her, what did you hope to get?
Q5   Why did you actually *hit* her? (instead of alternatives)
Q6   Did you think you were *right* to do this?

Q51   How do you think she felt afterwards?

We obtained answers to these questions with varying degrees of difficulty. Some men answered directly, whilst others would attempt digressions. We had to be very focused, which meant returning to the original question a few times. Some questions were relatively straightforward. For example,

Q26   Have you wanted to stop hitting your partner?

All men, without exception, indicated that 'of course they wanted to stop'. In order to challenge their commitment to change, we followed this up with the question:

Q26a   What have you done to try to stop yourself (using violence)?

This last question proved considerably more difficult for most men to answer, and suggested to them that simply 'wanting' to stop was not a sufficient commitment to prevent further abuse. When asking these questions, we sometimes made it clear that we were reading from a prepared questionnaire. By doing this we detached ourselves from the questions. If men had not responded to more direct probing, or if we judged the level of engagement to be too fragile, such questions lessened the risk of confrontation. Some men seemed more able to accept set questions than *ad hoc*, personalised probing. Of course, their receptiveness to set questions varied tremendously. Some were relatively open to challenge, whereas with others we barely penetrated the superficial responses. For example, one man made it clear right at the beginning of the interview that he would not be amenable to direct challenge:

> *R:*   You can forget this feminist claptrap if that's what you're gonna talk about. A man and a woman have got their place.

Maintaining power

The question of power differentials in research with men presents new questions for feminist researchers. Democratising the research process seemed completely inappropriate. We approached the interviews with the clear intention of *retaining* as much control as possible. Only from a position of relative control would we feel able to develop critical engagement and pursue different lines of enquiry. However, men were not always willing to relinquish or share control in an interview. We became familiar with a technique which a number of men used in order to acquire or maintain control. They would try to elicit personal information from us, presumably in order to divest us of the control we sought to retain.[12] For example, in the middle of a discussion about whether it was justifiable for one man to blame his violence on his drinking, he swiftly changed the subject:

R: Are you married?
I: Am I? No, I'm not married.
R: And do you think you're a dominant person?
I: What do you mean by that?
R: There's always one dominant person in a relationship really.
I: I don't know about that.

Retaining control was very important. Men's attempts to persuade us to disclose personal information were often designed to divest us of any power we did have, to suggest that, as people involved in intimate relationships, we must surely face problems similar to their own. Many men seemed to expect or want us to be similar in some way to their partner; some possibly used the same tactics to try to exert and maintain power and control.

We approached an interview knowing that men might try to manipulate or control us and were prepared to respond to such power games. Of course, not all respondents were ready to argue with any woman who stood up to them. Instead we sometimes found sad, lonely, depressed, inarticulate and passive men. Nevertheless, these men could, in very inventive ways, still attempt to manipulate the interview. When a man presents himself as very sensitive, fragile and guilty about his behaviour towards his partner, it can be extremely difficult not to indulge him or compromise yourself. Being beguiled by this subtle form of collusion can result in only minimal challenge and, though no obvious display of 'power' is demonstrated, the man is able to control the format and pace of the interview.

Similarly, men can disarm when they present themselves as plausible, charming and reasonable. Women often told us, as other researchers have been told, how others had disbelieved them because the public façade presented by their partner was so convincing. Again, this is a subtle form of power which can be difficult to deal with. Typically, those men who were eager to present as plausible were extremely resistant to challenge and were more likely to respond to probing questions by being hostile and defensive.

We do not intend to suggest that we approached every interview ready to question every articulation of sexist attitudes or beliefs. We could not question every minimisation or justification. We balanced the decision to question a comment with the degree of engagement we had established, with the time available for the interview and risk of antagonising the man. We had a fifty-page interview schedule to balance against a man's concentration span. Some men became uncomfortable with some of the questions and we used a range of cues to decide when to stop a line of enquiry – for example, facial expressions, body language, changes in tone of voice. At such times we might move on to alternative questions or move away from the interview schedule to talk about a less sensitive subject. We learned early on that many of the men we interviewed enjoyed nothing better than 'a good argument' during which they could demonstrate their (superior) knowledge and understanding of various issues. We sometimes had to disengage from such discussion leaving the man thinking that he had 'won', his attitudes thereby reinforced. Similarly, when we felt less able to challenge, some men may have interpreted this as our empathising with their explanations, justifications or excuses. We left these interviews disappointed, confused, frustrated. In the long term, we can justify these interviews in terms of the data we collected which contribute to the debate about men and masculinity and which will be used to develop feminist knowledge and understanding of violent men. However, these interviews troubled our consciences and remain as unresolved difficulties.

WHAT WE HAVE LEARNED

Hitherto, feminist research about men who use violence against women has explored *women's* experience of this violence. This has been a vital part of the campaign to protect women and children from men's abuse. However, by looking at the problem of men's violent and abusive behaviour from *men's* experience, we can start to build a new knowledge about men and masculinity.

We have been able to collect detailed data about an extremely sensitive and intimate aspect of men's lives. Our methods have enabled us to elicit a huge volume of information about men and their violence.

Not surprisingly, much of what we were led to expect from listening to women's accounts has been confirmed by listening to men. Men who use violence deny, minimise and blame. They do this to varying degrees; some are willing to accept some responsibility for their behaviour, others deny any culpability. Listening to men, it becomes apparent that their willingness to accept responsibility is closely related to their motivation to change. This is of crucial importance to practitioners working with violent men. The following are fairly typical responses of men who are far from willing to change. They illustrate just how entrenched some men's attitudes towards their partners are:

I: When d'you think it's OK to hit a woman?

R: OK? It's not OK but there's so much a man can take. It's just a reaction, he might just strike out with the back of his hand. If he's hit her, he's assaulted her, but maybe it was called for.

I: Why do you hit her?

R: Because I think she's deserved it – what she's said or the way she's said it . . . it's just one of these things that happens.

Similarly, we never ceased to abhor the full force of men's misogyny. Hearing men describe women as 'sly devious bitches' was grossly offensive to us. Communicating some of that feeling yet containing the depth of these feelings was often a difficult balance to reach. Although some men appeared to give us what they thought we wanted, portraying themselves as 'new men' who represented the paragon of equality in their relationships, others revealed to us their true misogynistic beliefs. For example, some men would rely on opinions about what was 'natural' behaviour for men and women, suggesting that violence on a man's part is an inevitable component of his masculinity:

R: Sometimes when you're a man you've got to take your aggression out somewhere. . . . I think every man's got it somewhere, unless he's a nancy boy. . . . It's the animal streak in all of us. It's the way God made us. You're better kicking a door than kicking a woman.

R: I've got to put ma hands up there and tell the truth. I'm no' very good at housework. . . . I wasnae born to be a woman. . . . I do ma share and I carry the heavy things and I get up every, *every* morning to get the kids to school. . . . Right enough, you might catch a 90's man wi his hands in the sink but you'll no' catch me doing it. It's no' ma place.

Our research methodology and interviewing styles have also enabled us to gather data about men's descriptions of their use of power and control over women. By adopting challenging techniques similar to those often used by workers on men's programmes, we have elicited from men accounts which, hitherto, have been absent from the research literature. Men who were willing to describe their violent and abusive behaviour in detail and who did not rely on denial, minimisation and blame were those for whom appropriate intervention could be extremely effective in bringing about changed atittudes and behaviour.

LOOKING TO THE FUTURE

Although it has often been gruelling for us to listen to men's accounts of why their partner 'deserved' to be beaten or how the violence was 'minimal' anyway, listening to men who are willing to admit the full extent and impact of their violence, take full responsibility for it and reveal a real commitment to change has been heartening. Hearing men's misogynistic accounts has been depressing, infuriating, frustrating, disgusting and heart-wrenching, but hearing others reflect on how they have changed and how they are committed to remaining violence-free, where this is supported by their partners' accounts, has enabled us to think optimistically about the future of relations between the sexes.

Interviewing men has not simply informed our understanding of how men perceive their lives; it has also developed our understanding of women. Many women wanted us to talk to their partner, to have the opportunity to see him as other than a wife-beater – for example, as a loving father or a good friend. In seeing these different facets of men, we could, in turn, appreciate some of the dilemmas women experience in making decisions about the future. Of course, other women wanted us to talk to their partner so that we might understand just how abusive they were. The experience of talking to men as well as women revealed to us just how complex and contradictory the nature of relationships between men and women are.

Listening to men talk about themselves, their lives and their opinions has also stripped them of some of the power which we had assumed they enjoy. Instead of seeing these men simply as powerful, we have also been able to see clearly that they too are disadvantaged by patriarchy. While their disadvantage does not involve the horrendous physical and emotional scars which women bear and can in no way be equated with the oppression of women in a patriarchal system, listening to them has brought home to us how their embodiment of masculinity requires that they live just half a life. In this form of masculinity there is no room for empathy, for emotional fulfilment through relations with another. There is space for only one ego, one person who dare not reach out to others for emotional support and company. The experience of interviewing violent men has reinforced our belief that men have much to gain from embracing an alternative form of masculinity and that, with appropriate practice, some men can achieve this. Most importantly, our experience has enabled us to reflect on how such research can form the foundation of a new understanding about men and masculinity which can be used to promote change in men through working with them to change their behaviour and attitudes.

NOTES

1 This chapter, although written by us, is the product of the work and energy of the whole research team. Rebecca and Russell Dobash, the Principal Investigators, have been a constant source of ideas, encouragement and support, and Pat Young, our Project Administrator, kept the administrative backbone of the project going with her consistency and patience.

2 We also interviewed 146 women. Interviews with women were an essential part of the project. Men's accounts of their abuse against their partners are often minimal and unreliable. It was therefore most important that women's accounts of their abuse be obtained in order to inform men's accounts. Though we will concentrate on the interviews with men, we will make reference to the women's interviews where appropriate.

3 Since 1968, probation work in Scotland has been the direct responsibility of the local authority Social Work Departments. Up until 1991,

funding of work with offenders had come from Scotland's five Regional Councils, but in 1991 the Scottish Office assumed complete responsibility for the funding of this work following the introduction of National Standards (1992 in England and Wales), which increased the priority of working with offenders and established guidelines surrounding such work.

4 See Chapter 3 by Monica Wilson for a fuller discussion of the CHANGE project.

5 For a fuller description of the research design and project generally, see Dobash *et al.* (1995b).

6 Whilst this notion of empowerment has been extremely influential in the feminist methodological literature, it is also more recently being regarded as simplistic. We cannot assume a common experience and shared understanding with all women. Messages of caution have come from other feminists who have been critical of researchers who intrude in women's lives and who expect too much from women respondents (Finch 1984; Holland and Ramazanoğlu 1994). Shulamith Reinharz (1992) has also warned of the stress placed on researchers by expecting all interviews between women researchers and women respondents to be an embodiment of sisterly love and support.

7 The project was funded by the Home Office, the Scottish Office and the Social Work Services group.

8 We had permission from the Sheriff Principal of Scotland to examine court records for the duration of the project.

9 It was essential that we obtain full accounts of women's experiences. This process of enquiry was an important aspect of interviewing women in terms of encouraging them to describe, examine and explore the content and meaning of their experiences.

10 The issue of interviewer gender is important here: many feminist researchers argue that it can be more difficult for male interviewers to resist colluding with men who use violence. We would argue that certain skills are necessary which can be acquired by either men or women interviewers: a good male interviewer is probably better than a bad female interviewer.

11 We did not take men's accounts as a reliable indicator of previous violence. We relied on women's accounts to provide us with a more detailed representation of the abuse.

12 Diane Scully (1990) notes how the men she interviewed tried similar tactics.

Chapter 7

Helping men to cope with marital breakdown

Jane Forster

SETTING THE SCENE

The year 1994, designated by the United Nations as International Year of the Family, saw an intensification of the debate about the family. Of particular interest to me in relation to work with men have been the spotlights that have fallen on fathers. For example, non-custodial fathers have successfully mobilised their fury to bring about changes in the policies of the Child Support Agency (CSA) – fathers can be angry, fathers can be powerful. The government has switched on its own spotlights, on the one hand emphasising the responsibilities of fathers through CSA legislation, on the other, refusing to endorse the European Community directive on parental leave, thus giving mixed messages about the role of men in families. The overall position of fathers in the 1990s has also been explored in conferences and debates. Edinburgh District Council's Zero Tolerance Campaign organised one such debate, posing the question 'Is there a future for men in families?' and concluding that men must do a lot of changing if they are to play a positive role as partners and fathers.

As a feminist, where do I find myself in these discussions? What was my motivation for undertaking a piece of social work specifically with men?

I came into social work with a primary interest in working with children. Their welfare has remained an important theme in my career. Valuing women as people in their own right was instilled in me from an early age, but feminist colleagues have played a significant role in encouraging me to recognise gender-based commonalities in the experiences of female clients, and connections between my life and the lives of my clients. Feminist perspectives were even more influential in helping me to make sense of the difficulties of empowering women while patriarchal structures, which sustain male privilege, remain so embedded in society. My more recent experience of working in a very hierarchical, male-dominated organisation has served to reinforce this lesson. My gender lens is sharper and stronger, my feminism is still developing.

In terms of social work's role within the family, I value the contribution that feminist literature has made towards exposing the extent of men's abusive, violent and controlling behaviour towards women and children in the family (Dobash and Dobash 1979; Brook and Davis 1985; Hanmer and Maynard 1987, Scully 1990; Langan and Day 1992). However, I cannot accept the radical position that sees no role for men in families or in the provision of public childcare (Pringle 1992). My personal and professional experiences challenge these perceptions and provide evidence of men who are not perfect but who are valued as partners and fathers. Such views are also supported within the literature (Hoyland 1992; Phillips 1993; Sharpe 1994). But then I have a stake in defending men – I have two sons. I identify with Angela Neustatter, feminist mother of sons, when she writes: 'I believe it vital that boys should be allowed to celebrate their masculinity, to enjoy physical prowess and to understand that in the eyes of their feminist mothers, their gender is not the worst thing about them' (*Guardian*, 20 September 1994).

Juggling the positive and negative perceptions of the contributions men can make to family life is important in reassessing the work that I undertook with men whose marriages had broken down. I did not embark on this work in the first instance from an explicitly feminist stance. I did it because I wanted to help the men and because I felt that helping them might have a positive spin-off for other members of the post-divorce family – that is, for the women and children.

My interest in working with men evolved from many years' experience of working with separated mothers and their children, and from active involvement in the development of Family Mediation Services in Scotland. Running through these experiences was an awareness of the significant role fathers continued to play in the lives of their families even after separation. As with the intact family, it was a role which could support and foster the well-being of the mother and child or which could act as a source of pain, instability and continuing oppression. There was also awareness of the fact that large numbers of fathers, estimated at about 40 per cent by research, would lose contact with their children altogether after separation (Jacobs 1982).

My interest was sharpened by a puzzle. Research had shown that men were deeply upset and troubled by the breakdown of their marriages (Hetherington *et al.* 1976; Wallerstein and Kelly 1980; Jacobs 1982; Ambrose *et al.* 1983; Jordan 1985). My own experience of working with families and knowing male friends whose marriages had broken down echoed these findings. And yet there was also evidence from research and my social work experience that relatively few men turned to social workers or counsellors for help. In Ambrose's study (1983), social workers tied with in-laws at the bottom of a long list of helpful people. Why should this be so?

The puzzle became a challenge. By learning more about men's experience of divorce and their attitudes towards social work and counselling, could a pilot service be set up which would be more acceptable and appropriate to their needs? In turn, by monitoring the pilot service, could we further develop our understanding of men coping with marital breakdown and our skills in working with them?

THE PILOT STUDY

I undertook the pilot project while I was working in Family Care, a small voluntary organisation based in Edinburgh which provided a well-established social work service for lone parents (mainly women) and their children. Staff in the agency were also involved in setting up community initiatives for women to develop approaches which built on ideas of mutuality and co-operation as an alternative to traditional social work models. The pilot project lasted for two years and, by the time I left Family Care, some fifteen men had been interviewed at least once, several had been seen on more than five occasions, and two had been in quite regular contact for over nine months. The men came from different social class backgrounds and were of varied ages, but could not be regarded as representative of British men as a whole. There were no men from minority ethnic groups. Nor did the sample include men who were referred because of an identified problem, such as child abuse or violence towards a partner.

Three factors emerge from the pilot and my subsequent experience of working with men which seem important for social workers to consider carefully when providing a service which is accessible and acceptable to men. First, we need to develop our knowledge base. In terms of my own project it was necessary to learn as much as possible about the impact of divorce on men, about relevant services and legislation and about men's attitudes to counselling. Second, based on this knowledge, social work methods need to be identified and skills developed which are appropriate to the needs of male clients. Third, the setting of the service – its location, image and staffing – especially if relying on self-referral, should be considered.

Knowledge and understanding

(a) The impact of divorce on men

In an earlier paper (1988), I summarised some of the research findings about the effects of marital breakdown on men – the effects on their physical and mental health, the effects on their work performance, the effects on their relationships with their children and with previous and future partners. Subsequent studies (Kruk 1989; Wallerstein and Blakeslee 1989; McCormack 1990; Simpson *et al.* 1993) have confirmed evidence of the upheaval caused to the men's inner and outer worlds, of their enormous sense of loss and of their being buffeted in seas of intense and conflicting emotions – yearning and bitterness, anger and fear, hurt and guilt.

While these studies paint a vivid picture of the effects of divorce on men, it was feminist analyses of gender relationships within the family which enabled me to understand more fully the significance of marital breakdown for some men, especially those who have not initiated the separation and those who become non-custodial parents (in both instances the majority of divorcing men). Hanmer and Statham (1988) review some of the research evidencing the power and control men exert within the family. Losing such power and control, as happens when a marriage ends, is likely to be traumatic, and men may feel themselves to be victimised by former partners and by legal and social systems, relating to areas such as custody, maintenance and housing. In their eyes, these systems may appear to favour the parent with children – that is, the woman. Thus, from the man's perspective, the power tables are turned, and some of men's disruptive behaviour in the aftermath of marital breakdown could be interpreted as an effort to reassert control or as punishment of wives who dared to challenge their authority.

(b) Relevant services and legislation

A complicating characteristic of marital breakdown for men and women is the fact that so many practical aspects of day-to-day living need to be sorted out, often in the midst of emotional and relationship turmoil. Information about relevant services and legislation is important for men in helping them to re-establish stability and with it, some sense of control over their lives. Receiving accurate, factual information from a social worker is helpful in itself, but may also play a key role in establishing the worker's credibility. For some men, receiving sound, practical help may give them the confidence to go on to broach more sensitive problems involving feelings and relationships.

(c) Men's attitudes to social work and counselling

A piece of my original puzzle was an awareness that men were generally more reluctant than women to seek social work or counselling help. In trying to understand what underlies this reluctance, I have drawn on my own experience and on studies of men and of male psychology. From experience, I know of men coping with marital breakdown who say they would not ask a social worker for help because they expect the worker to take their partner's 'side'. It would be easy to dismiss this explanation as a cover-up for other feelings but, just as we emphasise the importance of examining social work practice for evidence of discrimination against women, black people and those with disabilities, so it seems consistent to acknowledge that some practice could be biased against men.

Feminism has had a major impact on social work, and in recent years several writers have explored the development of a woman-centred practice (Hanmer and Statham 1988; Dominelli and McLeod 1989; Langan and Day 1992; Wise 1992). Underlying these developments has been an appreciation of the ways in which women have been oppressed by men, lending weight to accusations in some, mainly male circles, that feminists are anti-men. Such criticisms assume a uniformity amongst feminists which does not exist, while justifying rejection of feminism and social work along with it. For me, being pro-woman does not equate with being anti-men. However, I believe we do need to be careful that our feminist values do not colour our perceptions when we work with male clients. This may be especially so in the field of marital breakdown, where the raw edges of men's wounded relationships and feelings about women gape offensively. A skilled and experienced social worker, whose work I supervised, recognised this risk. She used supervision sessions to explore some of the difficult feelings that work with men aroused in her, and acknowledged that she had to concentrate much harder to tune into and understand the feelings and needs of some male clients, especially those consumed with hatred of women who had left them. At a more basic level, our conditioning from childhood onwards influences our attitudes towards men. Men are expected to be strong, to be rational, to take action. Men's behaviour following marital breakdown can be in marked contrast to these expectations. I recall two social work students, irritated and frustrated by their male clients who were trapped and immobilised by rage. The students found it difficult to perceive the underlying despair and hurt, and found it hard to tolerate men who appeared so helpless. It was as if this behaviour contradicted views of men which they were surprised to discover they held.

I have argued that there may be validity in the expectations of some men that social workers may be biased in favour of women clients, and that it is therefore important for us to explore and acknowledge our attitudes with honesty. However, I believe a more significant explanation for men's reluctance to seek social work help lies in understanding characteristics of men in general, and specifically of men coping with marital breakdown. Whilst I accept Segal's thesis that there is a 'multiplicity of masculine styles' (1990a: xi), common themes emerge from an analysis of male behaviour and from men's own accounts of their experience.

Three interrelated subjects are particularly relevant to understanding men's attitudes towards asking for help. First, men are status-conscious: maintaining status is important to most men. Tannen (1992) describes the ways in which this characteristic is evident in male communication, and explains how, when it comes to a situation where someone needs help (even help to find directions), 'many men, sensitive to the dynamic of status . . . are more comfortable in the role of giving information and help but not help in receiving it' (1992: 71). If men find it difficult to ask for directions to the bus station, how much more difficult is it for them to risk loss of status by becoming a client of a social worker? Crucial to a man's security of status is his need to be in control. As discussed earlier, when a man's marriage breaks down, his sense of control can be severely jolted and his whole being can feel undermined. Asking for help when feeling so 'male-fragile' is seen as an open admission of failure, and can feel like handing over the remnants of control to another person.

The third male characteristic concerns feelings. In most sections of British society men are brought up to hide their vulnerable feelings. Keeping feelings in check is part of being in control, and as a result, men are less likely than women to express or discuss such feelings. Rubin (1983), in a study of male/female relationships, summarises the socialisation messages which men receive: 'Boys are trained to camouflage their feelings under cover of an exterior of calm, strength and rationality. Fears are not manly. Fantasies are not rational. Emotions, above all, are not for the strong, the sane, the adult. Women suffer them, not men' (1983: 71). Rationality disintegrates when a relationship breaks down, and the eruption of intense feelings can challenge a man's sense of masculinity. The idea of going to a social worker or counsellor to explore these feelings is foreign to most men – 'how can just talking help? . . . and anyway that's the sort of thing a woman would do.'

Taken together, these psychological and social imperatives act to reinforce one other and may result in men retreating to familiar male strategies and behaviours (for example, drinking more heavily) in an attempt to rebuild a sense of identity. They may help to explain why so few men voluntarily refer themselves to social work or counselling agencies, and why those who do may arrive with very ambivalent feelings (Scher *et al.* 1987).

The service offered to men – social work skills and methods

In my social work practice, I have drawn on a variety of mainly individual approaches rather than specialising in any one method.

At times I have envied the expertise and conviction of specialists, whether they are client-centred counsellors, family therapists or task-centred practitioners, but I have also been wary of fashions in social work, which bloom and wilt or which fail to match the reality and variety of clients' needs. My experience of working with men coping with marital breakdown affirmed the value of being able to draw on a range of methods. My experience in the pilot project and work with men subsequently has sharpened my social work skills.

When I embarked on the project, I had read and been impressed by Wallerstein and Kelly's (1977) description of a divorce counselling service they had developed to help families. Based on their experience, they advocated counselling over a period of about three months, starting one to six months after separation and employing a variety of educational and social work approaches, depending on the needs of parents. They commented on the initial reluctance of men to be involved, but noted that there was often increased involvement as the counsellor's skills increased.

While Wallerstein and Kelly's work provided me with a framework, I soon found that I needed to be flexible. Men referred to the pilot scheme at very different stages in the separating process. Few fell into Wallerstein and Kelly's 'optimum period' of one to six months after separation. Whereas some came before separation, two came more than a year after, when they had started to emerge from a period of destructive, despairing behaviour, but could recognise how vulnerable they were to further setbacks. Their problems still revolved around the breakdown of their marriages, contact with their children and with the need to rebuild their own lives. My subsequent experience confirms my pilot observations that social workers need to be prepared to help men at very different points in their lives.

I learned to be flexible too about the length and focus of my involvement. Many men came only once or twice. The experience of social workers in my current work setting is similar. Within this 'brief intervention' group, I distinguished two main categories. First, those men who wanted information only – a contact name, or information about their entitlements. Second, there were those who were on the brink of an important decision – a decision to separate, a decision to visit children after a long absence, a decision to begin to socialise again. In the early days of the project, I sometimes failed to recognise the significance of the impending decision facing some men. Tuning in to the surrounding emotion and drawing on crisis intervention theory (Golan 1978), I saw the current predicament facing the men as an opportunity to explore unresolved, underlying issues. However, this led to men at times withdrawing from the discussion, and I quickly learned to change to a more problem-centred approach, focusing on the decision itself, exploring in detail alternative options and possible outcomes (Reid 1978).

With both these groups, it was often clear that the men were struggling with intense emotions and practical difficulties. Openings to go beyond the initial reason for the referral were only rarely taken up at the time. This was disappointing, but it also highlighted for me the importance in working with men of using the first interview as effectively as possible, recognising that it might be the only session, rather than the beginning of a longer contract. Several men did in fact return later, when faced with new problems, suggesting that the initial contact had been helpful, but also reminding me that coming to terms with marital breakdown is a long process. For men in particular, brief periods of counselling along the journey out of marriage may be a more acceptable and realistic option than a compact series of interviews.

Some men did use the openings to engage in longer-term counselling, and others were motivated from the start to explore their feelings and relationships, without relying on a need for information or an impending decision as a way in. In this latter group, it was easier to apply the approach outlined by Wallerstein and Kelly (1977) and draw on counselling skills. Thus I was able to help the men to examine feelings and relationships, both before and after the break-up, to assist them to deal with current difficulties and, in some cases, to help them turn from a preoccupation with the past to plan more optimistically for the future.

Practice issues

A number of recurring practice issues emerged which are relevant to work with men coping with marital breakdown, and most are relevant to work with men in general. First, it is important for the workers to clarify the scope and boundaries of their role early on and to be prepared to redefine these as work progresses.

Such clarification may allay some of men's ambivalent feelings about seeking help, and serve to reassure them that becoming a client does not mean abandoning individuality, independence and control. It may also be necessary to explain that the counsellor–client relationship is different from other relationships in their experience. As a middle-aged social worker, I was aware that I sometimes triggered memories of the men's own mothers, while two of the male workers found the clients latching on to introductory exchanges about sport and cars and had to resist invitations to the pub, the club or the football match.

But there is another dimension here. Most women social workers have had uncomfortable experiences of working with men, who may make very personal comments, with sexual innuendoes. The younger women involved in the pilot found themselves particularly vulnerable to such sexual harassment. I believe that sexual comments and attempts at friendship-building may be understood at times as examples of men trying to take control of the worker and to establish equal or superior status. At other times I believe this behaviour reflects their need to make sense of this new relationship by modelling it on more familiar relationships. Whatever the interpretation, I see the onus as being on the worker to explain and redefine the boundaries, while the responsibility to respect the boundaries is a shared one.

The second practice issue relates to the need to value male clients as people with strengths. Hanmer and Statham outline the principles of a non-sexist, woman-centred social work approach (1988: 140–3). Included in the list are the guidelines 'like women and enjoy working with them'; 'find ways of working that validate women's strengths'. Can we substitute 'men' for 'women' in these statements? This is a contentious subject, but I believe that if we are going to engage men and to work constructively with them, then we must try to do so. And yet how can we 'like' and 'validate' a male client as we listen to his account of his behaviour within his family and his criticisms of his former partner? It may be easier to empathise with the absent partner than with the client. By paying attention, do we risk colluding with the man and, as women, find ourselves hooked into traditional supportive roles?[1]

These are thorny issues which we all have to address. In spite of these ever-present dilemmas, on the whole I did enjoy working with the men involved in the pilot project and I found it possible

to identify and affirm the positive qualities which the men pos-
sessed. Thus, I took an interest in some of their skills, and encouraged them to talk about their jobs as bus drivers, furniture
restorers and factory workers, aware of the importance of work
to most men. I shared their pleasure when visits with the children
went well and their satisfaction, when as a result of careful fore-
thought, contact with their former partners had been constructive.
Enjoying, sharing and affirming, I believe, freed some of the men
to acknowledge their more negative characteristics; enabled
some to hold on to a sense of worth; and helped others to move
forward in their lives again.

The third practice issue centres on feelings. Even though most
of the men in the pilot study seemed to want to steer clear of
discussing their own feelings in depth, I still believe it is important
for workers to keep feelings on the agenda when working with
men, sharing with Bowl the conviction that 'it is often the social
worker who needs to show courage in battling against male inex-
pressiveness' (1985: 32). I sometimes made a point of checking
out clues to stress. How was he sleeping and eating? Did he
have any new health problems, chest pains, backache, stomach
disorders? Could he concentrate at work? Was he more irritable
with friends or colleagues? We discussed some of the research
findings about the stressful effects of divorce (Jacobs 1982).
Sometimes these approaches were helpful in opening men up to
recognising that their emotions were probably affecting their day-
to-day living. But sometimes I identified with Sharpe when she
wrote about the difficulty of getting men to describe their feelings:
'There were times in my interviews with fathers when I wanted
to shake them and say "Yes, but what did you actually feel
like?" ' (1994: 6). The area of helping men explore their feelings
is one in which more work needs to be done (Formaini 1990).

The final issue concerns relationships with significant others,
especially children and former wives, but sometimes parents,
friends and new partners. Research findings on the effects of
divorce on children emphasise the importance of parents explaining the reason for the separation; of non-custodial parents
remaining in contact; and of children growing up with a real,
rather than fantasy, picture of both parents (McCormack 1990).
With this knowledge, I felt that it was legitimate to introduce the
topic of children to the counselling agenda, and sometimes this
became an important focus of the work – discussing feelings

about losing day-to-day involvement in the lives of their children; encouraging fathers, when this was feasible, to establish regular contact; and helping them to understand the upsetting behaviour their children might display. Whilst I found it easy to be an advocate for absent children, I felt more wary of advocating on behalf of absent women. I was willing to explore ways in which the man might adapt his current behaviour to foster a better relationship with his former partner, or at least to avoid fuelling the simmering hostility. But I was reluctant to get drawn into taking sides in accounts of marital arguments, past and present, or to speak for a woman, whom I only knew through the words of her ex-husband.

On reflection, I think that my reluctance to intervene prevented me from helping some men to gain a better understanding of their relationships. A long-distance lorry driver in McCormack's study expressed the bewilderment of many other men when he said, 'I think the thing that shocks me most of all is that I knew so little of what was going on in my wife's head' (1990: 25). Social workers, especially those with a sound appreciation of gender differences, are in a good position to help men to understand the impact their behaviour and attitudes have on their partners.

There were times when I had a strong desire to stand up for absent women. In working with men coping with marital breakdown, some speak of their ex-partners in disparaging, sexist ways. Should we always challenge such statements? In principle, I want to say 'yes'. In practice, however, I prefer to attach qualifications, acknowledging that challenging others is not without risk. Some remarks are, of course, so offensive that a worker has no choice but to express disapproval and even consider terminating the involvement. But there are other times when I believe it is acceptable to exercise discretion and to assess the likely effect of challenging – would it detract from the focus of the work; would it threaten the relationship with the client; would it achieve its objective?

Once this assessment has been carried out, there is a place for constructive, sensitive challenge. For example, in working with a man who complained about his wife wanting to talk to him about her work at the end of the day, especially when she wasn't doing a 'real' job (she worked in an office, he did heavy manual work), I encouraged him to pause and re-examine his perception. He disregarded my challenge at this time, deafened as he was by the anger and bitterness aroused by his wife's leaving. However, several months later he was more disposed to listen, and I believe that some of the suggestions that emerged from our discussions, including listening to and showing an interest in a woman as a person, rather than as a sex object or potential housekeeper, may have helped him to lay the basis for more equal and respectful relationships with female friends.

The setting for the work

If we wish to offer a social work service for men, I think it is useful to consider where the service is located, how it is publicised and who staffs it.

I had no choice about the location for my work in the pilot project. Family Care is centrally located in Edinburgh – easy for men to find, discreet for men to approach and no one needed to know that they were visiting a social worker. Because the service was small and time-limited, it was not advertised, but instead I relied on referrals being made mainly by contacts in the Scottish Council of Single Parents, the Lothian Family Mediation Service and Parents Forever Scotland.

Ambrose *et al.* (1983) suggest that because men find it hard to seek help, the workplace is a good setting in which to both advertise and locate a service. My present employment with the Naval Family Service has allowed me to further my interest in employment-based counselling for men. It is clear from this work that some men whom we see as clients would not have approached a community-based social work or counselling service. There are, however, negative aspects. Men avoid the service, believing that referral will damage their careers; while social workers, especially when trying to challenge discrimination and male privilege, can feel oppressed working in a large, hier-archical secondary setting.

In addition to workplace counselling, men coping with divorce should have access to the existing range of specialist and generic services. This means that services must be advertised in accessible ways, and good links need to be established with other pro-fessional groups, such as solicitors and doctors, to whom men may turn first when their marriages break down.

Finally to the question of men or women workers. There is a diverse range of perspectives on this. Some acknowledge that men need help, but imply that they need to do this work themselves. Phillipson argues that 'Men need to work on their own understanding and behaviour and not expect or rely on women to help' (1992: 12). Seidler (1994) describes ways in which men have accepted this challenge. I believe that there is a place for women who wish to work with men. As women we have something special to offer, and the insights we gain from our work with men can enrich our work with women and children. Carlson (1987) describes the challenges and risks for women working with men, and emphasises the need to be firm and clear in one's objectives in order to avoid colluding with the male client, who may blame the worker, resist exposing his vulnerability and strive to hold onto power. Her overall message is that women can help men to deal with problems and, in doing so, help them to reassess their values and relationships, so that real and deep change is achieved. My own view is that both men and women social workers can be effective in helping men to cope with divorce and can learn from the skills and insights of each other, if there is open discussion of our practice from a gender perspective.

CONCLUSION

Sometimes in reflecting on my work with men, I have been struck by similarities between the experiences and needs of men and women coping with marital breakdown. Like men, women are often hurt and deeply distressed by the loss of a partner, and I have known women to react with vengeful anger, and castigate their ex-husbands and new partners, using abusive, sexist language. Men and women have much in common – good qualities and bad. However, this should not detract from the findings of research and feminist analyses which have highlighted real differences between men and women in the type and prevalence of problems, in the different meaning these problems have for their self-image, and in the social and structural context within which these problems are manifested. My own social work experience, in particular through involvement in the pilot project, has emphasised the value of understanding men's experience of marital breakdown and their attitudes towards social work, if we are to engage constructively with them.

Although I see my work as a beginning, with scope for further development and refinement, I am convinced that it is work that needs to be done. I believe that social workers have an important role to play in helping men to make the journey out of marriage an opportunity to reflect on their experiences, including the values and attitudes on which their family relationships were based, and to plan for the future with greater understanding of themselves and deeper awareness of and respect for other people in their lives. In turn this growth should be of benefit to their children, former wives and new partners.

NOTE

1 This theme is picked up in many other chapters, notably in Chapter 6, where Kate Cavanagh and Ruth Lewis argue that empathy with men is not possible, but that sympathy is, and that the key to feminist practice with men lies in the notion of 'critical engagement'.

Chapter 8

Sexuality, feminism and work with men

Cathie Wright

This chapter resulted from a conversation during which I talked about some of the difficulties and excitements of working with men on issues of sexuality. It is one thing to talk but quite another to write a clear exposition of the ideas and opinions that have arisen out of thirteen years of work in the field of sexuality and sexual health. In clarifying and defining what I have been doing and why, I have looked at what feminism means to me and how it relates to my work with sexuality and gender. I write as a practitioner, not an academic. My hope is that my observations might be of use to the reader in formulating new ways of viewing old questions. I offer this chapter as the starting point of a dialogue rather than as a definitive answer.

This chapter has a heterosexual bias because it is in heterosexual relationships that the most difficult issues arise between men and women. It is one of the most important arenas for male and female dialogue and conflict. I have endeavoured to communicate that much discussion about sexuality is common to all kinds of sexual relationships. I have chosen to discuss some aspects of sexuality that have arisen in my practice, and this means that violence and sexuality are not discussed at any length. It is a choice that reflects my view that there are many other aspects of sexuality worth considering which are seldom discussed professionally.

The chapter begins with an account of my view of feminism, followed by some discussion of sexuality generally and in relation to work with men. The latter focuses specifically on the development of my work with men generally and in relation to pregnancy counselling, sexual counselling and group work. Finally, I have tried to integrate the themes of the work in a statement about working with men.

MY FEMINISM

A key tenet of feminism is the value given to every woman's story, seeing each as a part of the wider political picture of women's lives. When I realised that my story with all its uncertainties and ambiguities was important and valuable, I was better able to hear and understand the stories of others. For me, the liberation of women is about 'Women demanding their full rights as human beings by challenging the relations between men (as a group) and women (as another) ... rebelling against all power structures, laws and conventions that keep women servile subordinate and second best ... women working consciously together for our rights' (Watkins *et al.* 1992: 3). My role as a social worker in this process is, first, to value women's experience and, second, to examine relationships between men and women from the woman's point of view. It is also to understand and challenge, and if possible, facilitate an alternative dialogue between men and women which respects and values their differences.

My current understanding of feminism comes from my experience as a woman and as a worker in the 'caring professions'. Only when I began to write this chapter, assimilating my political and professional experience with my personal life, did I realise the import of the early feminist statement that, 'the personal is political'. As the daughter of a liberated working mother, brought up in an all-female household, I never felt inferior to men and I found it difficult to relate to some of the early feminist debates. However, listening to friends and becoming more aware of aspects of my own behaviour made me realise that I too was profoundly affected by society's expectations of women, and that my problem in relationships were reflected in the experiences of other women. My experience was both unique but also shared by other women.

In my sexual relationships with men, I had to learn to disentangle lust, love and friendship, and at the same time attempt to understand why my expectations for an equal relationship were not being met. What I considered to be a dialogue was often seen as a threat to masculinity. My passions and concerns were trivialised. Such reactions I now see as part of the power struggle between men and women. At the time I was desperately hurt and puzzled. Only after many years did I realise that theoretical equality between men and women was limited by men's belief in their right to dominate and control women.

As I watched my sons grow up, the differences between men and women became more apparent, Tannen (1992), in describing the differing communication processes between men and women, argues that whilst the aim of much male communication is to exert power and control over others, female communication is more directed towards seeking connection with others. This made sense to me as I struggled with the realities of my family life. As I grew stronger and more assertive, I found that my relationships with men changed. I looked much more critically at the relationships of others. This was very valuable in my work and I became better able to understand both my frustration with, and my enjoyment of, male company.

Reading was a very influential aspect of my growing awareness of gender issues. Boston Women's Health Collective's *Our Bodies Our Selves* (1976), was an important text, especially in my work. Seeing women's views and experiences being recognised and valued in public validated my own. I also learned that women gained confidence and power by discussing aspects of their lives such as sex, masturbation and sexuality openly. Information and knowledge shared was also empowering. This philosophy became increasingly important in both my work and personal life.

My understanding of my work has progressed through a number of different phases. As a student I found that Freudian ideas made little sense to me. I was drawn towards action which ensured that people's basic rights and entitlements were maximised. I saw the social work role as having a strong advocacy function. As a generic, patch-based social worker, I observed that much distress arose from causes other than lack of basic rights. Emotional support and understanding contributed greatly to positive changes in the life style of my clients. Counselling and psycho-dynamic theory offered useful insights. At the same time I became aware that the majority of my clients were female, that they appeared to get little support from their partners and that they struggled against enormous odds. I realised, eventually, that only a feminist perspective helped me make sense of this.

My work with men involved a slow development of understanding about the attitudes and expectations men had of women and of themselves. I began to see men as vulnerable. I observed that in order to protect themselves they would exhibit aggressive and demanding behaviour. I became aware that many of my male clients felt quite unable to express the softer and more questioning side of their nature, and this made life for their partners extremely difficult. In my work at Lothian Brook Advisory Centre, I began to put together these strands of thinking. The needs of women were paramount because they were the principal client group, but I recognised that for women and men to develop more satisfying relationships it was important to work with both. It was simply not possible to ignore the needs of men, because in doing so I would be ignoring some of the major issues for my women clients. I needed to develop ways of working with men that did not deny my understanding of the position of women in our society. Poole suggests that, although men and women are different, 'none of the differences imply that one sex or the other is superior. Men and women are equal partners in humanity' (1993: 11). However, though we may be equal partners in humanity we live in an unequal society where men continue to exert power and control over women in all spheres of their lives. At this point in time, my personal and professional lives are turned to the same end, to increasing communication and understanding between men and women so that there is greater equality in close personal relationships.

SEXUALITY

In my work I have found that there are many different ways in which people use the word 'sexuality'. Some see it as synonymous with sexual orientation, others define it in relation to being 'sexy', whilst others associate it with the frequency of intercourse. Given this variation, some kind of common understanding of what is meant by sexuality, how it relates to sex and gender, is useful. I have developed a way of looking at sexuality from five different but related themes: the biological and physical base of sexuality, relationships, feelings, the social and cultural contexts and the spiritual aspects of sexuality (Burns and Wright 1993). It is logical to begin any consideration of sexuality with the body. Sexuality includes the act of having sex, it also includes gender, which can be biologically as well as socially defined. Sexual response is stimulated by ideas and fantasies as well as actual people and sexual contact, and it is firmly located in the body. The body feels sexy and, in the sexual act, follows a physiological pathway. Included amongst the five functions of sexual behaviour listed by Bancroft is the 'assertion of masculinity or femininity' (1989: 150). Bancroft suggests that an important function of sex is bonding in relationships between two people, often so that they can function as parents. Sexuality also plays a part in attraction between individuals whether the relationship be an overtly sexual one or not. We tend to like people whom we find attractive in some way, even though we may choose not to have sex with them. Sex in relationships can be used as a way of gaining power, of paying the rent or of inflicting pain. It can also be a means of expressing love, affection and intimacy for another person or persons. It must also be recognised that there are wide variations in human sexual relationships from casual encounters to lifelong partnerships.

However, managing both sexuality and sex in relationships is not easy. Humans have developed complex ways of managing and dealing with their feelings in relationships. Much of our theoretical understanding comes from Freudian ideas and humanistic psychology (Rogers 1951). It has been important to understand the effect of childhood experiences on adult behaviour. Understanding the way in which people protect and defend themselves is vital in helping with difficulties in all relationships, including sexual relationships.

Issues of gender and power are particularly important in sexual relationships. Masculinity is often defined in terms of activity and power, whereas femininity is often defined as involving passivity and submission. Behind that dichotomy is the fear of being vulnerable and weak, in itself a strong motivator for aggression. Sexual relationships above all are an arena for sharing vulnerability. It is not surprising that violence can be so closely linked with sex, but is is particularly dangerous because sexuality is so much part of our identity. Segal (1990b) describes the problem in relation to heterosexuality:

> The highly contested notions of 'gender' and 'sexuality' are at present conceptually interdependent. They are held together by the cultural imperatives and practices of a heterosexism

definitely linking the 'masculine' to sexual activity and dominance, the 'feminine' to sexual passivity and subordination.

(Segal 1990: 268)

Sexuality and identity are closely linked in the ways in which
individuals view themselves and their relationships, and in the
ways they behave. Sexual orientation is an important part of
identity, not only because it affects the choice of sexual partner,
but also because being in a homosexual or lesbian relationship
can be socially stigmatising. Thus identity is not purely a matter
of individual choice; it is also about how others define certain
kinds of behaviour.

Sexuality and identity are influenced by the way sex is
described and in the way in which stories are related in film,
television or print. Sex is seen as something to be controlled and
managed, and education, socialisation and religious traditions all
contribute to this. The cultural context in which we live affects
how we view our sexuality and our gender, though there is much
variation in how this is interpreted between generations and
across class, religious and racial boundaries. The many ways in
which gender differences are interpreted can have a significant
impact on individuals and their relationships.

Finally, there is a spiritual component to sexuality. This is sometimes difficult to comprehend; it links us with the wider cosmos.
It can be seen as using sexual energy to transcend bodily needs,
as in a celibate priesthood. The creation of children can be a
spiritual as well as a biological experience, and the sense of close
connection between two human beings can be a way of reaching
beyond the individual self. Spirituality can potentially involve
both good and evil.

Sexuality threads its way into all aspects of our lives, whether
or not we are sexually active. It is a force for pleasure but also
for extreme pain; the joy of good sex and the trauma of sexual
abuse and rape exemplify this. As social workers, we are in
constant contact with the difficulty and pain of others, and it is
essential that we have some understanding of our own sexuality
and how it has been affected by upbringing, gender, ethnicity,
class, and our own personal ways of adapting to life. Understanding ourselves is vital if we are to understand what is upsetting or
worrying for clients. This is particularly important when dealing
with sexuality, which touches on so many sensitive areas of life.

It is tempting to see sexual issues as too difficult and sensitive to raise with clients, but in my experience it can be immensely rewarding to open out discussion about sex and sexuality, showing that these issues can be discussed and understood, much as many other aspects of our life.

The issues that arise from sexual behaviour and which therefore present themselves to counsellors and social workers tend to include problem pregnancy, rape, sexual abuse and sexual problems, as well as relationship difficulties in general. Sexual orientation is often seen as a problem; it can be difficult to be open about homosexual orientation in a society which frowns on different expressions of sexuality.

Gender and sexuality are closely entwined. In intimate relationships the obvious differences between men and women are turned on their heads. For example, many men like to be both passive and active in sexual encounters and in their fantasy lives. Women do not always want to be passive. Men have expressed to me that their desire to penetrate is sometimes confused by their fear of being taken over and enveloped. Women have expressed a similar dichotomy, wanting to be penetrated yet fearing it. Such views have been expressed by both heterosexual and homosexual people, confirming my view that there is a duality in all of us which makes it difficult to adapt to the prescriptive norms of a society whose definitions of masculinity and femininity are narrow and restrictive. This is why there exist strong influences which encourage conformity exemplified by the opprobrium directed at people in public life who transgress the accepted norms of sexual behaviour.

Language often defines how sexuality and gender are perceived. In Scottish playgrounds 'poofter', 'slag', 'slut', 'cissy' and 'cunt' are current terms of abuse. Words for genitals and sexual behaviour carry a great deal of power, and when talking with clients it is important to check that they understand what is being said and are not offended by the worker's use of language. For many women, the most comfortable way of talking about their genitals is 'down there'; if they have a problem – for example, pain in sexual intercourse – they may have great difficulty in giving an accurate description of the problem. Their very discomfort is in itself an indication of their uneasiness with sexual issues. Men, on the other hand, have a much more 'friendly' relationship with their genitals.

In summary, discussions of sexual matters, though difficult, can be potentially liberating for clients. Sexuality allows us to express vulnerability as well as affection and warmth; it can be the vehicle for extremes of feeling, love and hate and destruction. The danger for workers is that they may only hear the extremes of sexual expression and lose sight of the normal and wholesome aspects of sexuality. In my experience it is only possible to contain these extremes by adopting a wide definition of sexuality and by understanding that sexuality, power and gender are integrally related.

SEXUALITY AND WORK WITH MEN

Development of work with men

When I joined the Brook Advisory Centre as senior social worker, I was interested in the difficulties that arise from sexual relationships. The bulk of my clients in the clinic were young women who usually came with problems involving sexuality or pregnancy. Sometimes they came alone and sometimes with their partners. Relationships between men and women were a constant theme for my women clients. In working with them, I began to reconsider what my role with men entailed. I saw, in a very raw way, just how destructive male behaviour towards women could be. I counselled women whose partners had abandoned them or forced them to have sex. I saw women who had been raped, some very brutally, and I felt angry and helpless in the face of this reprehensible male behaviour.

I also met men who were confused and uncertain, who wanted children when their partners did not, who tried to find a way of being human with the woman they loved. These men sought intimacy and close relationships just as much as women, perhaps more, as their friendships outside their relationships did not seem to give them the closeness they needed. The relationship with their partners seemed to be a source of status and pride, and often provided the only opportunity they had to talk about worries and concerns. Young women did not always see how important they were to their partners, possibly because they were never told. Some resented being the surrogate mother; disposable if the call of the peer group intervened.

I found that I wanted to stereotype men; to put them in boxes where their behaviour would be less confusing and difficult. I also found that I wanted to engage with men to help them get in touch with their feelings. How appropriate was this in feminist terms? Surely men needed to find their own means of self-expression? If women were to take on this role, how might they avoid playing traditional mothering and nurturing roles in the way women always have done, rather than developing more equal relationships which encourage men to take responsibility for their own actions? I pondered long and hard on these questions.

The advent of HIV/AIDS brought enormous changes to my work. When it became recognised as a sexually transmitted infection, sex education – and in particular, safe sex – received a much higher priority. The experience of working in a sexual health clinic had shown clearly the difficulties of condom use. For many years women had taken responsibility for contraception, subjecting their bodies to the effects of the pill and their minds to the fear of what it might do to them, though this was often seen as a fair trade-off for control over fertility. Men, on the other hand, had grown accustomed to leaving responsibility for contraception to women. It is ironic that HIV/AIDS with all its horror forced us to look again at sexual health issues, leading to more widespread discussion of sexual behaviour. HIV/AIDS meant a complete change in behaviour – first in requiring people to acknowledge the risk of infection and second in persuading them to accept and use the condom.

One approach was to try to remove the stigma of young women carrying condoms; to suggest that it was liberating for women to take care of themselves. The hidden agenda was that this was a back-up for those careless men who had lost or forgotten to buy condoms. However, in the end, condoms are only useful if worn by men, and this approach ultimately left the management of contraception with women.

A second approach was to encourage men consistently to obtain and use condoms in sexual relationships. This meant engaging with me either individually or in groups about their sexual behaviour; it meant talking about the mechanics of sex and the advantages and disadvantages of using condoms. What hindered this work was the behaviour of young men in groups and perhaps more fundamentally the ignorance of many male workers, and their consequent difficulty in talking effectively with young people about sexuality. They themselves needed to be convinced of the advantages of using condoms before they could be expected to communicate this effectively to others.

There is now a developing recognition that sexual health belongs to both men and women, and that both carry responsibility in relation to contraception and protection. In my present job, gender issues are seen as central, and both male workers and female workers are working conjointly to explore issues of sexual health with young people. At the same time, men have begun to meet together to talk to one another about sexuality and masculinity. Some of these men acknowledge their debt to feminism and are developing new ways of working with men.

Pregnancy counselling

Although the focus of my work at the Brook Advisory Centre was with young people and sexuality, counselling young women about their unwanted pregnancy and advising young women who were under sixteen about contraception were significant aspects of my work. The numbers of women attending the clinic who had been raped or sexually abused increased during the 1980s. I also saw men and women who were unhappy about some aspect of their sexual lives. The clinic was staffed by women and served a largely female clientele working together on issues of life, death and sexuality. It was a potent mixture which constantly raised uncomfortable questions for both worker and client.

As women spoke and I listened, I heard their questions and saw how confused they were about the men in their lives, and gradually I started to include partners more actively in the counselling process, especially where pregnancy was involved. However, from the outset, I had one clear principle: that women should have control over how the work was to be undertaken. The woman was the focus of my attention and she could choose whether or not her partner was seen; he was offered counselling because she wanted it; the power was with her. Women could also choose to see me on their own or with their partner or both. When I saw the partner I was interested in his feelings about the pregnancy and the relationship. I was particularly concerned that he was able to identify his feelings so that he could respond honestly, and not in what he may have thought was the 'right' way.

In this work, two very important statements were being made

which I see as fundamental to my feminism. The first was that women's experiences were valid and important. The second was that women kept control over the process as far as possible, the limitations on this control revolving around time limits on abortion procedures.

For men the procedure gave their experience and feelings value in a female context, with the woman having the power to choose what could happen to their unborn child, a significant and powerful political statement. The value given to women's experience in one context can strengthen the value they themselves give to it in other contexts. Likewise, the value given to men's feelings and concerns about their unborn child can have a powerful effect in validating their feelings. This practice offers the opportunity for honest and frank discussions to take place between men and women whilst at the same confirming the women's central position in, and control over, the dialogue and outcome. The following case-studies illustrate these themes.

Jane and Scott

Jane came to the Brook two months pregnant and aged sixteen, seeking confirmation of the pregnancy and considering an abortion. Her partner, Scott, was a year older and he came with her. Jane's parents did not know of the pregnancy and she did not want them informed because she felt that they would be both angry with Scott and disappointed in her. Initially, Jane had decided that she wished to terminate the pregnancy. She did not feel ready to have a child; she had plans for further education. She was aware that Scott was likely to disagree and felt very concerned about this. She was very much in love with him and feared his rejection.

Having spoken to Jane, with her permission, I offered Scott the opportunity to see me and asked him how he was feeling. He was bemused by such an enquiry but responded to the opportunity offered. He made his strong feelings for Jane clear and, whilst he was upset by the pregnancy, he was at the same time rather proud of his achievement. When asked about contraception he made it clear that he generally 'looked after' Jane. He either used condoms or withdrew before ejaculating. He did not see that there was any risk of HIV/AIDS because he was faithful to Jane. When I asked if they had considered contraception for

Jane, he replied that he did not believe in the pill because it would make her 'more available' to other men. His view was that if he kept control of contraception, he kept control of Jane. Similarly, he wanted her to continue with the pregnancy so that she would marry him and stay at home for him and the baby.

The final session with the two of them provided an opportunity to discuss what each wanted. In verbalising their individual wishes, each listened to the other and saw how far apart they were. Jane decided to have the pregnancy terminated and, whilst it was hard to see how Scott would cope with this and what would happen to the relationship, I felt clear that at least the process had allowed them both to express their views honestly in a safe context. If that opportunity had not been available I wonder how Jane would have fared? Would Scott have become violent, would she have been able to say what she wanted, might she have done what he wanted out of fear?

Catriona and Bill

Catriona and Bill were engaged to be married. Initially they had used condoms, but when they acknowledged their strong commitment to each other and a wish to be faithful to each other, Catriona began taking the pill. However, during the previous month she had been sick; the pill had not worked and she was now six weeks pregnant. Both were nineteen and in their first year at college. They were very uncertain about whether or not to have the pregnancy terminated. Catriona asked Bill what he thought. He replied that it was her body and her decision which he would ultimately support. Catriona was furious; she felt Bill had opted out of the decision. She wanted to know what he thought. If he disagreed with her, she knew it could affect their relationship and she did not want her decision cast up at a later date. Bill did not know what to say; he felt he had no right to influence her decision because it was her body. He found it hard to acknowledge that it was half his child. Space to consider his position was important for both of them, and finally he did say that on balance he thought termination was the best option. The relationship was, however, severely shaken by this experience, because Catriona felt that Bill had not really supported her in having to be persuaded to comment on something they were both responsible for.

These two cases raise several issues. First, procreation is a powerful urge for both men and women. When a women looks at her life, children may have given her a role and adult status. She may want to focus only on her children, but increasingly she may expect to continue to work and derive status and satisfaction from both children and work. For a man, a child may mean a similar confirmation of manliness and adulthood, but his life is unlikely to be focused on the children in the same way as his partner, though this has changed in the last decade. Both may see children as restricting their freedom. Conversely, children may be *the* most important part of their lives around which their family life revolves. All this is a reminder that some men have strong feelings about having children, despite those others who appear to avoid all responsibilities.

Second, underlying both these situations is the question of whether or not to seek abortion, and who has the ultimate responsibility for making that decision. In law, it is the woman's body and the woman has the right to choose whether or not to have the pregnancy terminated. It has been a central tenet of the feminist movement that women should have control over their bodies, and this has included the right to choose when to have sex and whether or not to have a child.

Third, the two cases also illustrate two couples coming to a decision about a pregnancy in which the woman has the final say, but the process by which she arrives at that decision is often complex and can involve the participation of a partner. We cannot on the one hand criticise men for not facing their responsibilities as fathers whilst at the same time deny the reality of conception. Both parents can have important roles in a child's life.

The role of feminism is to redress the balance of power. Women are no longer the chattels of their husbands and have responsibility for their own lives. Yet, overall, men have more institutional power, more earning power and take more power in their relationships. They are generally physically stronger than women, which in sexual relationships can mean non-consensual sex. To redress the balance means to encourage women to speak out, to express their views, and to claim equal value and power in partnerships and sexual relationships. This also means creating a forum in which men can hear the concerns of women, so that they can begin to change their attitudes and behaviours. Men also need opportunities to express and understand how they feel, and then to understand the implications their views have for women. From such a dialogue, change is possible.

My observation of what goes on between men and women when pregnancy and abortion become issues suggests that there is a great need for men to admit they have feelings and to identify openly and honestly what these emotions might be. Women tend to express how they feel verbally, whereas men often act out their feelings. Redressing this imbalance is important. Women and men need to understand each other's point of view but men need to be able to express what they think and feel about relationships, intimacy and sexuality. Women have a role to play in this. I see my work as facilitating this development of under-standing by allowing that dialogue to take place.

I also believe that this dialogue is more difficult for my male colleagues to conduct. Many of the women and men I have worked with have intimated that they would find working with a man more difficult. Given that women are expected to listen and support both one another and men, it is not surprising that many of my clients have felt more comfortable talking to a woman. From this standpoint, women can begin to develop new under-standings about men. We must remember too that what also legitimates feminist work with men is a recognition that women want us to work with the men who are often a very important part of their lives.

Sexual problems: sexual counselling

Work with men and women on the particular difficulties of their sexual relationship often illustrates most vividly the differences and conflicts between male and female expectations and experi-ence of sexual expression.

Men and women are both literally and figuratively naked and vulnerable in their sexual encounters. Sexual counselling involves exploration of the most intimate aspects of relationships. It often has a strong educational component. Workers must have a sound knowledge of sexual issues to enable them to get to the heart of the matter quickly and effectively. In order to reach that point, it is necessary to have done some personal work on sexuality so that responses to clients are not negatively affected by our own discomfort. This does not mean giving up strongly held views about, for example, sexual morality, but it does mean being self-aware, recognising that others may have different views. Clarity about the purpose of intervention is important so that personal opinion is clearly recognised and only expressed in order to support the client in the work being done.

Sexual counselling also includes discussion of sexual practices and feelings, so it is important that workers are comfortable with the language of sexual expression and are able to talk confidently and explicitly about sex. The ability to respond in an unembarrassed way can reduce anxiety: acceptance and a sense of humour are also important aspects of effective sexual counselling.

The educational components of such counselling may focus on contraception, or disease, but it is more likely to be specifically about sexual arousal and response. For example, men are often ignorant about female sexual response, and are therefore not always aware of the effect of penetrating a woman when she is not properly aroused. Women are often uncertain about male arousal, feeling that they 'cause' erections and therefore must 'do' something about them, or their partner might suffer deeply from frustration. Explicit discussion of these matters is very important in validating the experience of men and women in helping them understand their difficulties with intercourse.

The two most common male problems are erectile dysfunction (impotence) and premature ejaculation. Both are very threatening to male identity and are closely linked with anxiety about performance. Women may not understand why their partner is unable to give satisfaction in the way that they have been led to expect. In such cases, sexual counselling can help men understand their difficulties and reassure women that the problem is not necessarily their fault.

Reactions to these sexual difficulties are determined by the ways in which the individual has developed sexually and the significant influences on that development – for example, family attitudes and responses to sexual expression. Men and women are sometimes brought up to view sexual behaviour in very stereotypical ways. Happily, many of these views have changed enormously over the last two decades. For example, the initiation of sex used to be the prerogative of the man and this often allowed him to control any sexual activity. Women often had to sacrifice their desires and find other ways of meeting their own needs. However, not only are more women proactive in their sexual relationships, but it is also more acceptable for both men and women to express themselves in ways previously regarded as gender-specific'; women can be dominant, men can be passive. These opportunities, while liberating for many women, can be very threatening to men and some respond by withdrawing from sex, in much the same way as women once did. Counselling men around sexual problems involves identifying and exploring the numerous ways in which they can behave sexually and which may give satisfaction to their partners. For some men this can be very liberating, but for others removing the masculine blueprint for sexual behaviour is very difficult. Many fear that they may not live up to their partner's expectations; many feel very vulnerable in sexual relationships. Managing that vulnerability is a crucial part of the process of dealing with sexuality in relationships. It is erroneous to assume that men do not seek intimacy, though the ways in which they achieve closeness are rather different from those of women.

A further aim of sexual counselling is to foster some kind of mutual understanding between couples of the different ways each of them approaches intimacy, taking care to acknowledge any fear they may have in this area. The aim of such counselling is to improve the relationships by encouraging men to be more aware of themselves, their inhibitions and their fears.

Sexual problems: group work

Group work with educational objectives often illustrates most vividly the differences and conflicts between male and female expectations and experiences of sexual behaviour. It offers opportunities to examine and reconsider sexual relationships in ways that might lead to change.

My experience in counselling young people, both couples and individuals, has informed the work I have done with groups. I have focused on the need for information as well as the importance of encouraging the development of personal awareness around gender and sexuality. A central theme has been my awareness that, at the deepest level, men and women seek closeness and intimacy. Group work offers a unique opportunity to encourage discussion of these issues, whether in single-sex or mixed groups. I have worked as a sex educator with young people, as a trainer of workers who work with young people and staff groups who work with, for example, drug users, people with a physical disability, and people with learning disabilities. My focus with all of these groups has been sexuality and how to feel confident in discussing it.

Workers who lead such groups should have undergone some form of experiential training to develop their personal self-aware-ness, as well as having group-work skills. Ideally, groups should be led by two workers, one male and one female. In recent years I have become increasingly positive about working with young people in single-sex groups, especially when the focus is sex edu-cation, as long as there are opportunities to move into mixed groups at a later stage. I have found that both young men and young women value the opportunity to talk in same-sex contexts about sex and sexual relationships. They are more likely to use these sessions constructively and less likely to dismiss, criticise or ridicule each other. Once they have had this opportunity, they often feel able to talk more confidently, honestly and respectfully with those of the opposite sex.

Generally it is easier to work with young women. They are more in touch with their feelings and often better able to articu-late them. Group work with young women can be very stimulating and rewarding; their motivation to participate is high and dis-cussion can be extremely wide-ranging. However, groups of young men tend to be harder to motivate, and without firm direction, the discussion often degenerates into 'banter' filled with sexual innuendo and derision. However, if one of the group leaders is female, then this banter is more restrained, and the discussion more focused. For this reason I think it is very important that women are involved in this work with young men. When the leader is male, my concern is that worker and men are more likely to collude with each other and that sexist behaviour and language are subjected to less challenge by the male worker.

As a worker who is concerned to tilt the balance more fairly towards respecting women, I have wondered in the past if I should leave work with young men to the male workers. I have since concluded that this work should not be left to men. I believe that training and continuing group work has a very important role to play in opening out the discussion so that men and women together can identify the important issues and learn from each other. When women are involved, they can not only identify but also challenge discriminatory behaviour from workers and men. This role is not an easy one for women to adopt but I think it is essential. Group work of this nature should be informed by women and their experiences, and women should have some influence over both content and practice to ensure that challenges to sexist behaviour and attitudes are continually presented.

Another question I have struggled with concerns the roles adopted by women in working with men. Are we drawn into adopting the maternal role, leaving male workers to talk about sport, for example? And what about male workers working with young women? On balance, I have come to the view that it is helpful for male workers to do some work with young men on particular issues such as male relationships, in which they can offer role models to young men. This can encourage more openness and new ways of behaving and relating to each other. However, I believe it is critical that male workers receive training on gender issues and sexuality and that the lessons learned from feminist work are incorporated into the development of their own thinking and practice.

I was very powerfully affected by co-leading a group of young male social work clients with a male colleague. It felt as if I was being allowed to watch something rather private which belonged to a different way of being. I was nervous about my involvement in this group. I felt middle aged, middle class and very aware of being female and different. I decided to dress 'up' for this group, almost underlining my age and status; I think this gave me confidence. The group ran for four two-and-a-half-hour sessions, over a period of four weeks, and aimed to develop the participants' knowledge and awareness of sexual health. This was undertaken in stages and included a number of different activities which enabled the participants to look at different aspects of relationships and sexuality – for example, friendship, romance, homosexual and heterosexual relationships, the language and biology of sex.

If I felt odd in the group, it was quite clear that the participants were not quite sure how to respond to me. If one of them made a sexist remark (consciously or unconsciously), then they looked at me anxiously to see how I would react. They did not say anything that caused me offence; if they had I would have responded firmly, though taking care not to denigrate any individual. Neither did they indulge in the man-to-man banter about women which might have prevented serious consideration of the issues. They found the discussion on language particularly difficult, but it was also the point at which they started to relax and felt able to ask basic questions about female sexuality. Once they heard some of my views and realised that I could cope with their way of talking about sex, they felt able to speak more freely.

The last session of the group was particularly enlightening. They all spoke openly and honestly about themselves and their experience. We talked at length about responsibility for contraception and the risks of HIV/AIDS. I was struck by their frankness about how hurt they had been by women who had rejected or laughed at them. I could also see how their roughness, ignorance and lack of understanding would have caused pain to their partners. It opened out a new world of male confusion, vulnerability and pathos. Most surprising of all was the extent to which the male workers and clients shared this ignorance and lack of understanding of women.

Looking back, my presence provided the female dimension. This was vital; from my observation it prevented extreme displays of sexist language and behaviour and encouraged the group to focus on what, for many, were extremely difficult issues. My male co-worker was able to open out different ways of being male and this allowed me to relax and listen to what they had to say.

CONCLUSION

Many women spend a lot of energy trying to work out how to live with men, and we as workers need to be attentive to that concern and struggle. The feminist perspective enables us to contextualise women's lives; our understanding and challenge of men's struggle to find balance and satisfaction allows for the possibility of change which can lead to better, more egalitarian lives for both men and women.

There are basic differences between men and women which provide the spice and challenge that make the relationship between men and women interesting. There are fundamental similarities in the need for love and intimacy which should be valued. Recognising both similarity and difference is important in understanding sexual relationships and their problems. Both men and women can be very vulnerable in the sexual arena and this means that they can both behave in defensive and destructive ways. Understanding that vulnerability will help to challenge the defensive behaviour which can so often destroy what is most important.

Chapter 9

Building fragile bridges
Educating for change

Rowena Arshad

In preparing to write this chapter about working with men on issues of equity and rights, I read extensively hoping to find material which I could readily absorb in order to move the debate on. It came as a surprise that there was so little recorded and published about feminist work with men generally and particularly in relation to social work. There have many publications on the roles of men and women in social work, on the effects of men on women, women working with men in caring professions, men's opinions about men but a dearth of literature on the actual issue of women working with men to construct an anti-sexist framework for practice. This chapter records my experience as a Black[1] woman trainer on anti-discrimination issues and my work in that field with male colleagues. This chapter could be described as anecdotal, but every discourse needs to start somewhere and therefore I make no apology for drawing heavily from the personal.

IN THE BEGINNING

I was brought up by my mother. My parents divorced when I was four, and I was the only child. In the country where I grew up, divorced women were viewed with a mixture of pity and fear. Pity because they did not have the backing of a man behind them and fear because they were viewed as a threat to the relationship of other couples. The country where I grew up did not operate a welfare system and I was conscious throughout my childhood of how hard my mother worked to support me. My father, disappointed because I was a girl, took no interest in me and provided my mother with no financial support as I was growing up. I was aware that despite the multiplicity of roles women had, their status, like many women world-wide, was nevertheless secondary to that of men. I grew up within a culture of orthodoxy which labelled me as a child of a divorcee. When I came to Britain in 1977, it was with rose-coloured spectacles and high expectations for my future. Perhaps naively, I did not anticipate finding discrimination and injustice here. My awareness and consciousness were very quickly raised but mostly in relation to my colour, not my gender. My early experiences of racial prejudice and racism affected me in many significant ways, contributing to my understanding of oppression and its diverse forms. The gender issue paled into the background as the issue of colour moved gradually to the fore.

My early influences came from the Black movement with the works of women writers like Amrit Wilson (1978), Angela Davis (1981), Hazel Carby (1982), Wilmette Brown (1983), Swasti Mitter (1986), bel hooks (1984, 1989), and Harriet Jacobs (1988), to name but a few.[2] These writers challenged the notion that 'sisterhood is powerful' arguing that the term 'sisterhood' can also be misleading unless contextualised. Writers like Anthias and Yuval-Davis (1983) sought to problematise the notion of 'sisterhood' and the implicit feminist assumption that there existed a commonality of interests and experiences amongst all women without recognising the existence of diversity. Black feminists have argued that, within the feminist debate, issues which might appear universally relevant for all women have specific meanings for Black women. Carby (1982) questioned the general applicability of concepts such as 'reproduction' 'patriarchy' and 'the family' just as hooks (1984) sought to redefine feminist theories of work, violence, sexuality and parenting. Stacey (1993) also highlights the ways in which power differentials between women and men are further layered by differences in power between women depending on where they are positioned with the histories of racism, colonialism and imperialism (Afshar and Maynard 1994).

Stacey's (1993) comments are crucial to this chapter because my experiences of being Black within a white Britain has affected the way I work with men and how I locate myself within the women's movement in Scotland. Like many other Black women I would agree that the family can be a source of oppression for women (Barrett and McIntosh 1982), but it also serves as a refuge for many Black women (Bhavnani and Coulson 1986). I find my family unit is often the only security I have in the face of negative and often hostile experiences, yet I fully recognise that sexism does shape my private life and intimate relationships. The convergence of these two contradictory aspects of my life is the setting from which I see, experience and make sense of the world.

Whilst it needs to be recognised that Black men benefit from patriarchy, racism, both individual and institutional, ensures that Black men do not have the same relations to patriarchal, capitalist hierarchies as white men. Racism requires me to forge alliances with Black men in a way white women do not always need to with white men. The words of the Combahee River Collective capture my point – 'we struggle together with black men against racism, whilst we also struggle with black men about sexism' (Moraga and Anzaldua 1981: 213).

For many women, it is not a simple task to talk about men. Within a patriarchal society, the voices of women are rarely heard. Whilst many have been ignored, many others have been silenced or indeed silent. We have been taught from an early age to be uncritical of our fathers. First-wave feminist writers and activists raised awareness of the ways in which women's lives and experiences had been ignored. They also challenged many of the stereotypical ideas and attitudes about women. Women not only began to articulate and reflect on their experiences, through collective practices such as consciousness-raising, they also developed a critique of men which has continued virtually unchanged since the rise of the women's movement in the 1960s. Some feminists (hooks 1984) have highlighted women's hesitancy to discuss the issue of men, and many feminist activists are still reluctant to critically explore the issue of working with men or to generate a discourse about feminist strategies for the transformation of masculinity, viewing such work with much scepticism. However, fourteen years of New Right domination should spur us on to realise that as feminists, if we are to locate and make explicit the nature of our arguments and strategies for change, we need to be the producers of the text.

My journey to understand and articulate the processes of discrimination and inequality stem from my daily diet of racism. In predominantly white Scotland, being Black affects my life chances more significantly than being a woman. However, as my capacity for critical thinking has developed, so has my realisation that I cannot divorce the 'woman' part of me from my colour, class and age, and I have learned to make the connections across them all, thereby giving voice to the varied dimensions of my life. The notion of separatism has therefore been alien to me. My practice has always been based on a model which asserts that issues of inequality and powerlessness are best challenged through collective action and open dialogue. Dominant themes are those which address the redistribution of power, the encouragement of community action, the promotion of local control, an understanding of structures and a reliance on networking, collaboration and solidarity among those who are disempowered. Framing this 'radical' model are my distinctive experiences of being Black and a woman (Bourne 1983).

I do not always operate within the radical model of practice. In reality, most of my practice probably takes place in the blurred areas between theoretical models. Given that ideological differences exists between different model of practice, being an 'eclectic' practitioner is not without its difficulties. As a Black feminist whose political philosophy is grounded in socialism, I recognise that traditional socialism has marginalised the contributions and needs of women and Black people. The subordination of sexism and racism to class has also produced difficulties which are not always easily resolved (see Hanmer and Rose and Petruchenia in Thorpe 1985). Cockburn (1991) suggests that all strands of feminist theory – that is, liberal, radical and Marxist-socialist – have been and remain equally valid and that most feminists are a little bit of each. My own thinking and practice reinforce this view.

WOMEN AS TRAINERS OF ANTI-DISCRIMINATORY PRACTICE

Most anti-discriminatory trainers recognise the existence of a variety of dilemmas which confront us daily in our work. The purpose of anti-discriminatory training is two-fold. The first aim is to raise practitioners' awareness of the dominant themes within the equality debate and the legislation which underpins practice within Britain, and the second is to enable changes within practice to take place through the provision of opportunities to examine and reflect on the issue of equity and rights. As the drive for competence-based education and training persists, the challenge to trainers is to recapture the meaning of education so that anti-discriminatory practice is not reduced to the demonstration of technical competence. In anti-sexist training, my role is to broaden the discourse; to enable both men and women in the group to begin to explore the root of the problem as well as the symptoms. The process is as important as the outcome.

For the last three years, I have been involved in offering anti-racist and anti-discriminatory training to social work colleagues. In the ten years prior to that I worked with other groups in the statutory and voluntary sector as a trainer in anti-discriminatory practice. When I work with a group, it is generally a full day session and my agenda is open and declared. By this I mean that participants are aware from the outset that the training session has been designed to provoke thoughtful discussion on discrimination issues. Attitudes and language will be open to question and the key task is to work towards raising awareness and facilitating change through honest and open dialogue. The audience is not always sympathetic. On the contrary, many of those attending trainings courses are resistant, some having been instructed to attend by their employers. Groups are generally composed of both men and women, though seminars for senior managers tend to be predominantly male whilst those for children's centres are almost exclusively female.

I always begin by informing participants that we are here to explore and learn rather than judge and condemn. Participants are assured that examining concepts like 'equality' and 'discrimination' is both conceptually problematic and open to much individual interpretation. They are encouraged to think of the day as a valuable opportunity to learn, to reflect and to develop critical awareness of the processes of discrimination. The question of 'political correctness' is raised, and participants are assured that it is better to be honest and open throughout the day than to engage in politically correct verbal cleverness. Mistakes are allowed as long as learning follows. The main aim is to open up dialogue, with the hope that from dialogue will come change. Change is important and necessary. Much care is taken to construct an atmosphere of openness and honesty. Attempts are made to narrow the gap between trainer (expert) and participant (learner) and much effort is put into encouraging a positive, safe and constructive learning environment (Humphries 1989).

As a Black woman trainer, several dilemmas confront me as I carry out my work. I am conscious from the outset that I am different. Very often, I am the only non-white person in the room. I wonder if the participants will see me primarily as a trainer, or will it be my difference they notice first? I am aware that being Black increases my visibility but this difference does not give me high status. As a member of a minority group, I am the focus of many of the stereotypical ideas and attitudes associated with Black people. This visibility adds pressure: I often walk a tightrope wondering if my competence will be noticed or if participants will be too busy just noticing the difference. I find that people have high expectations of me as a Black Asian woman trainer and consequently I have to work harder to prove my productivity and credibility.

But being a Black woman can also mean being in vogue. Some participants would view the difference as being sufficient reason to legitimise anything I said. I am expected to be a 'culture expert' and to fill those I train with knowledge about ethnic minority communities. In addition, as a Black woman trainer, I recognise that I spend much energy refuting the stereotypical judgements often made of Black and female trainers. For example, I try to be extremely articulate and patient, aware that many white people believe that some Black people tend to go through life with a 'chip on their shoulder'. These are pressures which my male white trainer colleagues do not have, although they argue that I can claim 'colour and gender' credibility which they lack. Some of my male colleagues assert that as white men involved in anti-discriminatory training, they are less likely to be taken seriously since they do not speak from lived experience of discrimination. Unfortunately, they do not always recognise the pressures that being the 'token Black woman' generates, either. Ethnic and gender status in anti-discriminatory work can be an asset in a few circumstances but a trap in others. It is often difficult to remove the tag of cultural expert. Further, other competencies and skills often go unrecognised and unappreciated. I often wonder if my employers recognise the totality of my ability or whether they court my presence because I am their token cultural asset.

TRAINING MEN AND WOMEN: SOME DISTINCTIONS

'Citizenship is to do with belonging, becoming a member' (Allen 1992: 132). This need to belong and to blend is not an uncommon response for most people. Within the groups I work with, as with any group, the desire to feel accepted by those you are working with is very strong. Being a trainer differentiates me from those being trained and this difference can threaten both trainer and trainee. If I choose not to assimilate, this can threaten an audience, and any subsequent discussion or activity on my part, however reasonable, may be viewed as problematic.

However, in an all-women training group, one important aspect of the assimilation process disappears in that there is shared commonality in gender. I find I behave differently within an all-women group than when I am in a mixed group. Within an all-women group, I am generally more relaxed and more confident in dealing with issues of racism and discrimination. Challenges are less likely to be confrontational. However, when men are present, this confidence changes. If they are men who are politically 'aware' of equality issues, I relax and behave as I would in an all-female group. If they are resistant, my confidence in being able to maintain a conducive learning environment generally weakens. I have identified three explanations for the differences I have experienced in training men and women. First, men are unaccustomed to being challenged and censored. In situations where their practice or professionalism are open to critical comment, there is a greater tendency for them to resort to behaviour that undermines others in the group, including the trainer. Such behaviour includes the use of verbal cleverness to attempt to outwit or score points, employing reductionist strategies which relegate every debate into 'hard facts' – if it is not statistically proven, it is not valid. For example, if I cannot prove there has been an increase in racial attacks in the last few years, the problem must be less urgent than I have suggested it to be. Women participants on the other hand tend to accept that no statistical increase in racial attacks could be explained by low reporting levels. Other undermining strategies also include the use of diversionary tactics such as monopolising the debate, thereby silencing the remainder of the participants, moving the discussion onto another subject or criticising the relevance and applicability of the material under discussion to their work and lives.

The most undermining type of male social work colleague is one sometimes referred to as the 'anti-sexist sexist'. This is the man who is knowledgeable about gender issues, who uses the language of equality but whose attitudes and behaviour towards women continue to be discriminatory and oppressive. He is often conscious of the fact that he is white and male and therefore in a powerful position. He subtly communicates this message to the group, thereby reinforcing his own position. He will often dominate discussion and can be a beguiling participant whose views are deferred to by the other participants, who may feel threatened by his apparent knowledge and grasp of the issues. His super-consciousness actually begins to oppress the group. I have a range of techniques for coping with such men. For example, I may ask them to identify some central aspects of their theoretical framework and then I will use their own examples as a basis for examining their behaviour in the group or I may ask them to give space to others in the group. However, my concern is that these men, although engaging on an intellectual level with the principles of anti-sexist practice, manage skilfully to deflect further critical scrutiny of their practice. Left unchallenged they might contribute to changes on the margins of power but the central tenet of male dominance remains untouched.

Second, just as men are unaccustomed to being challenged, so women are unaccustomed to doing the challenging. Throughout my growing-up years, I have subliminally internalised the message that women should be around but silent. This discordance within myself does affect my self-confidence in mixed-sex settings. However, I now consciously encourage women to question and challenge not only the men in the group but also one another.

Third, in mixed settings, as a Black woman, I can never be sure if any potential racial prejudice within the all-white group will be more powerful than the force that should technically unite me with the other white women in the room against sexism. Men in general tend to dominate group discussions either verbally or by body language. By contrast women colleagues engage in shorter contributions and are generally more apologetic than their male colleagues.

REFLECTING ON MY OWN PRACTICE

Having mentioned that men tend to dominate discussions within training sessions, I have been conscious that I have allowed this to continue, especially if the contributions have come from male colleagues who are aware of the processes of discrimination and can contribute usefully to the discussion. I have been conscious too of allowing these men more speaking time in the hope that through them others in the group will learn. This can mean that other participants, often women, have less time to speak. I find such situations difficult. As a feminist, I believe it is imperative to engage in constructive discussion with women colleagues within an all-women setting and the lack of opportunity to do this is frustrating. Doing this work confirms not only the rich diversity of women's lives but also their different level of awareness and understanding of gender issues. Many women need space to discuss and understand the personalisation of the political in their lives and the politicisation of the personal. Many find this difficult in mixed settings. Consequently in such settings, whilst I am building alliances with those who are aware, I have to be careful not to alienate those who are not, particularly if the latter are women. In all settings, I endorse women's presence, their experiences and womanhood generally.

I now work with each group at the beginning of a training session to set ground rules. One of those rules is respect for one another. Another is giving one another time and space to speak without being interrupted, ridiculed or marginalised. These 'rules' are negotiated and agreed by all present, and adhered to. I also monitor how often I interrupt participants and try to ensure that I do not give less weight to either the contributions of women or those less aware of the issues.

WOMEN TRAINING MEN: THE MALE PERSPECTIVE

Difference is not difference to some ears, but awkwardness or incompleteness.
(Trinh T. Minh-ha, quoted in Giroux 1992: 226)

Rationale of the research

I spend a significant part of my working life training men to be more aware of their sexist behaviour and the societal, institutional and personal attitudes, values and ideas which underpin this. One of my primary objectives is to provide opportunities for men to consider critically the nature of the relationships which exist between men and women, taking into account issues of power, control and oppression. As the feminist struggle has progressed and as feminist critical consciousness has deepened and matured, it is now acknowledged that the reconstruction and transformation of male behaviour is a necessary and essential part of the feminist revolution (hooks 1989). Thus, after twenty years of the women's movement, we might expect to find that men's attitudes and behaviours have changed. As a trainer, I hope to contribute in some way to that change. Therefore, in gathering data for this chapter I decided to write to the men I had trained recently in order to elicit their views and share some of their perceptions about sexism and gender issues.

I conducted a small-scale study of the men who had participated in the anti-discriminatory training courses I had conducted during the previous twelve months. These courses were either distinct modules within a number of social work education and training courses (Diploma in Social Work, Scottish Vocational Qualification Programme). I opted for a short questionnaire as the data-gathering instrument, and whilst I recognise that the use of questionnaires raises questions of reliability, validity and representativeness (Gilbert 1990; May 1993), it seemed an appropriate way of gathering information in a relatively short period of time.

The research questions fell into three categories. First, I wanted to explore what men thought of the issue of sexism generally; second, I wanted to ascertain their preference on the issues of mixed or separate sex-training settings; and third, I wanted to offer men the opportunity to proffer their thoughts on issues of anti-sexism and gender. I was also hoping to reflect through some of their answers upon my own effectiveness as a woman trainer of men on anti-discrimination issues; does training help men to develop their understanding of sexism?

I sent out 46 questionnaires and received 27 (59 per cent) completed returns. The analysis which follows is of these 27 responses. I hope that some of the issues raised through this small survey will be of use to colleagues within social work in articulating questions which might also be of concern to them. It will also be of use to trainers of anti-discriminatory practice.

Profile of respondents

Of the returns, 93 per cent were in full-time employment, the others being students on training courses; 89 per cent were between thirty-one and fifty years of age. All were white though classified themselves in a variety of ways from European, Scottish, Irish to WASP (White Anglo-Saxon and Protestant). Eighty-five per cent of the men indicated that they did not consider themselves to have a disability. Eighty-six per cent trained within Scottish institutions: all were social work trained having attained either the CQSW or the new Diploma in Social Work and 63 per cent completed that training between 1986 and 1993. This is significant in that it was during the mid- to late 1980s that many professional associations and local authorities began to incorporate policies and procedures designed to eliminate discriminatory practices in all their various forms. The new Diploma in Social Work (CCETSW 1989) also appeared, promoting anti-racist practice and anti-discriminatory practice. Therefore it would not be unreasonable to expect men who qualified during the late 1980s and early 1990s to begin to reflect an understanding of the processes of discrimination. It is surprising to note that 60 per cent of the respondents had no prior experience of anti-discrimination training before the session I ran. Of the returns, 67 per cent were from men who classified themselves as managers whilst the remainder were students, lecturers and training officers. This picture reflects the predominance of men in managerial positions within social work and the current under-representation of women in decision-making within the higher echelons of the profession, well-documented in the social work literature (Howe 1986). Seventy-eight per cent of the men worked for Scottish local authorities, whilst the remainder worked in higher education or the voluntary sector. Workplaces ranged from residential homes for children, young people and the elderly to mental health teams.

Awares of sexism

The men were asked to respond to questions designed to elicit their views of sexism. All of these men were prepared to acknowledge an awareness of discrimination against women in the home and in the workplace and the majority were supportive of anti-sexist initiatives. Given this level of awareness and support, why then is a significant amount of anti-sexist practice from men not immediately evident? One simple explanation for this finding is that some of my respondents may have told me what they think I want to hear. I have no way of confirmimg this but I prefer to take a more optimistic stance and view these data more constructively in an attempt to ascertain what, if anything, women can learn from it.

It is this discordance between theoretical support and practical action that needs to be addressed. The task of connecting theory to practice, of ideas to action, remains the inevitable chasm that has yet to be crossed by so many of us, both male and female. Vic Seidler (1991a) warns that sexism is not simply an abstract ideology that has to be challenged in people's heads but is a complex set of social relationships that is lived daily. He suggests that it would be easy to create a false dichotomy, whereby men are involved in the 'psychological' changes through consciousness-raising but women remain the forces for change in terms of structural discrimination. Men may demonstrate intellectual commitment to anti-sexism through a mixture of verbal cleverness and emancipatory ideologies, but how many of them have been at the forefront of campaigns which challenge structural change on the basis of gender? Many have been very involved in campaigns which attack class inequality because of class and capitalism but how many have linked this to the effects of patriarchy both publicly and personally? Seidler's concerns are supported by many women (Hagen 1992) and some men who acknowledge that, whilst men may pay lip-service to women's demands for change and equality, in reality 'feminism was just a mirage on the horizon.' (Carpenter, quoted in Chapman and Rutherford 1988: 14). Many pro-feminist men (Bowl 1985; Hearn 1987; Morgan 1992) have warned against a politics of rhetoric without an interrogation of masculine practices.

Transforming sexism entails rethinking the issue of gender and reliving the contrast between private and public (Gamarnikow 1986). This means more than just lip-service from our male colleagues and partners about 'justice' and 'equal opportunities'. Faludi asserts that 'when the issues change from social justice to personal applications, the consensus crumbles' (1992: 81). However, my own results do indicate that there is a glimmer of hope that our male colleagues in social work are perhaps searching for a dialogue and ways of effecting change. As a trainer in many fields other than social work, I believe that professions which seek to empower individuals, and which are (if rather recently) committed to anti-discriminatory practice, have the essential values on which an anti-sexist movement can be built. I have no doubt that the men who responded in this survey are not representative of public opinion but perhaps their consciousness has been shaped by the value base of their profession.

Ability to recognise and challenge sexism

The next theme follows on from the above discussion. Whilst all of the men said they were aware of sexism, they were also asked to comment not only on their ability to recognise this discrimination but also on the ways in which they actively challenged this. Ninety-six per cent felt they were able to and did both recognise and challenge sexism. However, whilst I cannot know whether this is translated into practice or remains an academic notion, the result is optimistic. Some respondents commented extensively on their views of sexism and masculinity. One offered his understanding of why many feminists were sceptical of contemporary men's groups, 'Men's groups are as old as history itself, rules of the ancient Greek city states etc . . . all bastions of patriarchy. Women therefore have good reason to be suspicious when they see men getting together. After all the usual result is drunkenness, violence and misogny.'

Another respondent went on to say: 'I believe it is crucial for men to support women's struggles while recognising that it is also crucial for them to take responsibility for themselves, which means engaging critically with those men who seek to defend what they take to be their rights.'

A few men commented that whilst some men wanted to engage in debates about redefining masculinity, women had to recognise that men too were operating within a patriarchal structure and ideology which some found oppressive. One man acknowledged that women were sick and tired of supporting men in their efforts to change. He felt that any discussion of sexism exposed vulnerabilities and had to be conducted in a safe atmosphere where feelings could be shared and reflected upon. He felt that challenging sexism was central to men's reconstruction of their maleness adding that it was a constant repudiation of the 'feminine' which held masculinity firmly in its place.

Such responses suggest that if feminists are to reconstruct the text, we need to work with such men to create a new paradigm where old dialogues are not simply recycled or added to but are replaced by a new language and greater understanding. This new dialogue would encourage the challenging of language, behaviour and attitudes as a central means of moving towards a society that is less oppressive to women.

Biology versus social construction

Only 55 per cent of respondents were of the opinion that gender was socially constructed; 45 per cent viewed gender and gender differences as 'natural' or 'biologically' determined. This was a disappointing finding. In practice I have found that those attending training courses frequently assume that gender is based on inherent characteristics. The nature-versus-social-construction debate (Pateman 1987; Ramazanoğlu 1989) seems to retain its appeal and the arguments about male strength versus female domesticity appear to have retained their resonance. Perhaps more alarming is that the tenor of the discussion has become more sophisticated. After two decades of the women's movement, we assume that few men and women today subscribe wholly to the notion of biological determinism as a means of explaining gender differences. Many of us accept that much of our perception of gender roles has been learned and reinforced through male-dominated structures, practices and language. Yet within this small sample group, 45 per cent still felt that gender differences were 'natural'. What this signifies is the huge move still required to shift thinking beyond biological categories.

Writers like Shulamith Firestone (1979) began the debate by arguing that the oppression of women by men is rooted in biology, thus pre-dating and overriding hierarchical structures based upon economic and social relations. Firestone asserted that women's liberation lay in acknowledging women's essential biological differences from men and that it was important that women revalue the creative and nurturing aspects of their femininity which had become devalued or distorted in partriarchal society. Others (Pateman 1987) are critical of such Hobbesian reductionism and similar argument which ultimately can be used to assert that women's subordination is decreed by nature and is therefore immutable. Pateman (1987) argues that it is necessary to develop a feminist theoretical perspective that takes account of the social relationship between women and men in historically specific structures of domination and subordination. Feminist theories have to explain the ways in which patriarchy has shaped and dictated the multiplicity of roles women have had over centuries, both in their public and private lives. However, genetic arguments appear to have become fashionable once again as scientists of the New Right attempt to utilise biological arguments to explain personality traits and other supposed inherent characteristics (Wilson 1994; Quest 1994). My research leads me to suggest that in the future I must include the biological arguments in training if only to allow for their public refutation.

The gender debate: mixed groups or all-male groups?

The majority of respondents (67 per cent) expressed a preference for mixed sex groups, believing that a mixed group would allow for debate and sharing of views and experiences. Some felt this was vital in shaping frameworks for future action. Two respondents felt that all-male groups would not be challenging enough and that men were so deeply conditioned into gender roles that sexist attitudes might not be recognised within all-male settings. Some felt that any discussion around sexism needed to be informed by women's experience and opinion, acknowledging that in mixed-sex groups women are often held responsible for initiating and developing the discussion. Women are often used as the catalysts of change; it is often expected that their experiences and analyses will be exposed in order to facilitate men's learning. If we want to influence how men challenge sexism then, I believe, we have to be there when the dialogue is taking place and at times act as teacher and guide. After all, if we insist that future action must be grounded in the reality of women's lives, then women have to be the checkpoints. The role of women in educating men is complex and the cost to women can be high. Men must take responsibility for their own behaviours but women have a role in helping men see differently. Women in mixed groups discussing gender issues need to differentiate between those men who want to gain knowledge to assist their struggle against sexism and those whose interests do not go beyond intellectual curiosity or even those who want to find out about women's perceptions so that they can more effectively counter feminist arguments. After a decade of working in the area of attitude change, I am more able to differentiate between these different men, using a combination of pointers – for example, the ideological framework that informs their arguments, the consistency of this with their practice, their ability to link different issues of oppression, their body language, mannerisms, choice of working terminology, the way they work with other women in the group. Other women, I'm sure, have identified similar indicators which can be useful in their work with men, always remembering that useful indicators can never be absolute guarantees.

Of the respondents, 11 per cent indicated that they would prefer an all-male group. The basis of this was the need for a safe group where men had the opportunity to meet to discuss how to reconstruct their masculinity. One respondent felt he had gained much positive experience in all-male groups especially when it involved discussions around sensitive and controversial issues like sexuality, sexual abuse and male and female roles in society. Yet another stated that he felt that an all-male group should be accountable to women, especially on issues of sexism. This relates to previous comments made about the need for male groups to be informed by women's experiences. One respondent in this category preferred an all-male group because he felt that women, often guided by strong feelings, may take discussions too personally. Such views reflect men's overwhelming ignorance of the reality of women's lives and confirm the continuing existence of traditional reactionary views of women.

Among the respondents, 18.5 per cent stated that it did not matter if the issue was discussed in a mixed or all-male forum. One respondent had been part of an all-male group for two years and felt that all-male groups were useful to assist in the exploration of personal feelings around very sensitive issues such as sexuality. However, he also indicated that a mixed group would allow for more focused discussion on sexism and the action needed to challenge sexism.

Modification of behaviour during training

This study asked if men participating in anti-discriminatory training modified their behaviour during the actual training sessions.

I included this question in the hope that anonymity would provoke a truthful reply. If male respondents did modify their
behaviour, several conclusions might be deduced from this. First,
they were sufficiently aware of the gender debate to differentiate
between those behaviours and views which were acceptable and
those which were not. Second, men change their behaviour when
there are women about. Third, men modify their behaviour within
safe situations where they do not expect to be ridiculed. It could
be one or a combination of these reasons that resulted in 41 per
cent of respondents indicating that they did modify behaviour.
Interestingly, the majority of these were men who demonstrated
a higher degree of awareness of gender issues through some
of their other answers. This perhaps enabled a higher degree of
critical self-reflection when answering this question, thereby evok-
ing a more honest reply. Another 26 per cent said they did not
know if they modified behaviour but some within this group felt
that the mere acknowledgement of this fact was in itself difficult.
The other 33 per cent said they were always conscious of their
behaviour and language regardless of setting.

Two key points to emerge from the answers to this question
were that men can change and that they were most likely to do
so within a safe environment where admission of their sexism is
met by constructive dialogue rather than ridicule. Some comments
from the respondents illustrate these points.

> Men can quickly feel constantly criticised, judged and con-
> demned and become defensive and retaliate.

> The media may periodically have fun knocking contemporary
> men's groups and this in part further increases stigma attached
> to the idea of men meeting together to talk about issues like
> masculinity and relationships with women.

> I believe that anti-discriminatory training sessions *can* provide
> the safe spaces that men need to begin a dialogue with each
> other and with women.

**Should women trainers be involved in anti-sexist work with male
colleagues?**

The majority of men in this study (64 per cent) said they would
feel more challenged in training sessions run by women. Many

felt that men rarely challenged other men on issues of sexism unless there was a woman present. When women are involved some men are encouraged to feel that their challenge might be supported by the women in the group. Others describe the importance of showing solidarity and building alliances with women. Not only is there is a degree of patronage associated with these points but also the motivations underlying the latter in particular are somewhat disconcerting. Surely anti-sexist stances by men should not be about scoring points in front of women? It was also felt that some men regarded challenging sexism as something of a game to be played but not to be taken too seriously (by men at any rate).

Some men suggested that women who challenge sexism do so with more conviction. The frequency of challenge was also mentioned. Men were of the opinion that they challenged discriminatory practice on a more *ad hoc* basis, whereas women were most likely to present consistent challenges to sexism. This is an interesting finding for, whilst some men regard women as more likely to challenge sexism than men, my own experience suggests that many women feel uneasy about challenging some types of sexism when they encounter it.

Two respondents did recognise that women trainers tend to be tentative in challenging male attitudes for fear of entrenching those attitudes. Both described this approach as unhelpful, and suggested that a strong, assertive (rather than aggressive) approach would be most effective in working with men on sexism. This is a reminder to all feminist trainers and practitioners to be confident in ourselves, our principles and our intentions and not to be apologetic for having a democratic vision.

Learning points from the research

There are several pertinent points to emerge from my study. First, all of the men were aware of the existence of discriminatory practice and were, at least theoretically, supportive of anti-sexist intiatives. However, many still depend on the presence of women to either take the lead in anti-sexist work or to motivate men to give this work a higher priority. Second, the majority of men in this study stated that they felt more challenged by women in the area of anti-sexism, and just under half indicated that they did modify their behaviour when participating in anti-discriminatory training. They acknowledge that women bear more of the responsibility for tackling sexism. Very few men (18.5 per cent) in this study were familiar with feminist writings and fewer still (7 per cent) were familiar with men's writings in the area of masculinity. The reluctance of some men to explore alternative theoretical frameworks which offer different ways of 'seeing' and 'being' is disappointing though not surprising (Alcoff and Potter 1993). Power is not easy to relinquish. If changes are to occur, then more men need critically to examine masculine practices and the ideas which underpin them and translate such knowledge into positive action which challenges oppression against women. A reluctance to scutinise and analyse is possibly one reason for the inaction, apathy and confused practice demonstrated by many men, leading to men's continued abdication of their responsibility in working to end sexist oppression. Fear of being vulnerable, fear of censure and ridicule by other men are also possible reasons. However, many men are committed to feminist ideas and principles (Jardine and Smith 1987) and have endeavoured to push back the boundaries. Cockburn (1991) states that men gain hugely from patriarchy and men's opposition to women's liberation is, therefore, on the face of it, nothing if not logical. If men were to act it could mean qualitative and revolutionary change in their lives. Another reason for men's resistance to change, she asserts, is that men too are entangled in the reproduction of patriarchal relations.

The most encouraging findings to emerge from this study is that many of the men who participated acknowledged the existence of sexism. This recognition, although minimal, is fundamental if change is to occur. For an anti-discriminatory trainer, this awareness is a necessary first step for any man if he is going to begin to challenge inequalities and discrimination. However, it is not only feminism that challenges men and disrupts current notions of masculinity and femininity. Transformations in the economy and political structures are also necessary.

WORKING WITH MEN: TOWARDS A RADICAL FEMINIST PRACTICE

The following are some points which I think feminist work with men must also consider.

First, any educative work with men must include the recognition of the ways in which sexism affects men and women personally (the individual level of thoughts, feelings, attitudes), culturally (societal perceptions, assumed shared ways of seeing, thinking, doing, cultural folklore, humour) and structurally (the institutionalised forms of discrimination, the way discriminatory practices have been woven into the fabric of our structure). Power, politics and struggle are at the heart of any feminist work with men. In our work with men, we must never lose sight of our feminist framework which acknowledges clearly that women unlike men are hostages to systematic institutional oppression through sexist ideology (Barrett and Phillips 1992).

Second, anti-sexist work with men must be informed by the lived experiences of women who are the disempowered within patriarchy. Giving voice to women should not be solely about sharing different women's experiences but about giving meaning to the voices so that men can begin to understand them. It is not about relating accounts of victimisation but rather about using such experiences to analyse and identify ways in which men can begin to redress some of the power imbalance.

Third, work with men must be grounded in a keen sense of the importance of constructing a vision for revitalising democracy for both men, women and children. Our approach cannot be reduced to forcing men to pledge an allegiance to anti-sexist principles. Through discussion and exploration with men, we can begin to create relationships and structures where the notions of difference and equality are reconciled with the imperatives of freedom and justice.

Fourth, a radical approach must focus on the issue of difference in an ethically challenging and politically transformative way. This will involve feminists in developing their understanding of the ways in which men's identities are constructed and reproduced, acknowledging the anxieties that men from all social strata are facing as the processes of market philosophy push each of us deeper into a web of consumerism, individualisation and confusion. We need to move beyond 'blaming' men. Eardley states that

> we think that in the current crisis – or rather, accumulation of crises – the far right's new 'toughness' has an attraction for men who are in confusion about a role that is being progressively undermined. . . . The left's hesitancy on these questions

means that many men have 'nowhere to go' except to be more conservative, more divided, more protective of tiny areas of privilege, looking after number one.

(Eardley 1991: 138)

A gender under siege begins to develop a siege mentality, reverting to what is familiar as a form of self-preservation. It is therefore important that feminist workers do not apply another form of prejudice by guilt-tripping men; this merely sends the perpetrators underground. A comparison can be made with the racism awareness training (RAT) movement of the early 1980s. The RAT model promised that, through a process of critical self-reflection, white people could begin to redress some of the wrongs they had perpetrated on Black people. By attacking the consciences of individual white people many became further confused or came to resent the whole anti-racist movement. Sivanandan (1985) warns that whilst the RAT approach encouraged white people to own their racism, it failed to address wider structural discrimation. Unless the root causes of individual problems are located within a social, economic and political context, individual problems will be seen as having individual causes and solutions. Many of the issues we are dealing with such as domestic violence, sexual harassment and lack of childcare provision, are issues which cannot be solved merely at individual level. Any anti-sexist work needs to be located within a framework which challenges the distribution of power and works in solidarity with men to dismantle patriarchal structures.

Fifth, I would argue it is crucial that we know the framework from which we are operating when working with men. Plant suggests, we should aim to 'explore a meaning: before we espouse a cause' (Plant, quoted in Martin 1987: 12). Working with men is becoming popular and more and more people will contribute to this discourse. As feminists we need to know why working with men is important for us. We work with men because we want to improve the quality of life for women, to allow space for dialogue to take place where men can hear from us and us from them. We write about men to enable a reconstruction of the text which allows critical insight gained from feminist perspectives to shape the discourse so that the text and the practice which follows are informed by a politic of solidarity that humanises and liberates both men and women. Unless men and women converse and begin to understand each other's anxieties and frameworks there can be little movement in transforming gendered productions systems which continue to oppress women (Ramazanoğlu 1989). It is therefore heartening that a large majority of men in my study preferred to address issues of sexism and gender equality in mixed groups.

Sixth, we must work to create communities of interests and communities of resistance. As Cockburn states, 'patriarchy is not the only relational system governing western societies. Gender relations are lived as class relations. Class relations are gendered' (1991: 221). Recognising the specificities of other forms of oppression is necessary; this helps us to understand how different oppressions interact and reinforce one another, forming a totality of oppression which is often extremely difficult to penetrate. (Ramazanoğlu 1992) suggests that 'men are to be empowered through the reconstruction of women rather than to be rendered helpless or destroyed' (1992: 184). It is on this basis that the feminist voice will continue to have resonance. A separatist approach can only be counter-productive. Separatism does not preclude the right of women to choose only to work and live with women but their political struggle will need to encompass women and men for the sake of all our futures.

CONCLUSION

Challenges to power invariably produce resistance in one form or another. New Right ideas dominate the political spectrum, and values and ideas which reduce the autonomy of both men and women into functional units for the purpose of market and profit are glorified. Ramazanoğlu (1992) reminds us that we cannot afford to be Utopian about the prospects for women's liberation when we live in a precarious world system dominated by private greed, competitive individualism, economic crises, sectional and international violence, increasing poverty and environmental disasters. At the same time we must not forget that men – our male colleagues, our fathers, sons and brothers – are also caught in this same system. We must acknowledge the men who take on the challenge and work with feminists to dismantle the patriarchal framework. We need to open up space for dialogue and disagreement. Lessons must be learnt from the anti-racist movement where white and Black are, to quote the old cliché, learning to 'unite and fight'. Campbell (1994) reiterating a point made by Baldwin, asserts that if we are prohibited from talking about a problem it doesn't simply go away. It lurks in the background, like a corpse hidden in the cupboard. When people visit, all of our attention is focused on what's behind the cupboard door and this prevents us from talking about anything useful. I believe it is important to ensure that feminist practice never relegates work with men into such a cupboard.

NOTES

1 I have chosen to use the word 'Black' with a capital to denote that it is used as a political term to include all people of colour who suffer racism.
2 Many of these names are still not familiar in mainstream social work.

Chapter 10

Working with boys

Gilly Hainsworth

HISTORICAL BACKGROUND

From its beginnings in the second half of the nineteenth century the youth service has defined the needs of girls and boys as entirely different. Then, as now, the primary targets of the service were the poor urban working class, who were, and still are, regarded as being in need of particular guidance to prevent their becoming, in the case of boys, dangerously criminal, and in the case of girls, morally degenerate. The service was intended to extend the moral values of the middle and upper classes who funded it and to a great extent ran it, to these 'at risk' young people. For girls this generally meant providing Bible study and training in how to serve and to excel in the domestic arts. For boys a rather different agenda was operating. Any leisure time that they might have was seen as a potential hazard to the community, and there was a pressing need to 'keep them off the streets'. William Smith, founder of the Boys' Brigade, stated the aims of the organisation as being 'to promote habits of obedience, reverence, discipline, self respect and all that tends towards the Christian manliness' (quoted in Davies 1986: 93). To this he could have added the need to foster jingoistic patriotism and pride in the British Empire. Working-class lads could be needed as cannon-fodder in a potential war, and had to be kept in a state of readiness: competitive and aggressive but obedient and loyal to the Establishment.

Pearson (1983) argues that the emergence of the notion of adolescence as a distinct social category in the late nineteenth century must be placed in its political and economic context, and understood as illustrative of the desire to institutionalise middle-class child-rearing practices. Children who had earned a living street trading were stigmatised at this time as delinquent, though it was not so much their behaviour that had changed, but rather official reaction to them.

The growing labour movement gave little attention to 'youth', its focus being rather on 'workers'. It perceived the division of young and old as reactionary, when solidarity and unity of purpose was the desired outcome. So youth work was left to wealthy philanthropists and Christian organisations, including the Girls' Friendly Societies and the Young Men's Christian Association, and was relatively untouched by any radical or progressive movements for almost a century.

The Second World War brought women out of their homes and into the workplace, raising women's political awareness and their expectations. Although post-war propaganda may have attempted to reverse this trend, women's presence in the public arena had been established to such an extent that this trend was now irreversible. In the years after the war, feminists and socialists shared a platform to fight for the creation of a welfare state, believing that, in it, many of the old antagonsisms – between middle class and working class, and between men and women – would disappear (Taylor 1983). The idea that women should be entitled to share public spaces with men filtered into youth work in the 1950s, with mixed youth provision becoming more prevalent (Davies 1986).

The post-war period also witnessed the development of a new partnership between the state and its citizens. There was a new acceptance of the role of the state in intervening in the lives of individuals and families. This is evident in legislation on everything from secondary education and health provision to the Children Act of 1948 (Seed 1973). In 1960 the state finally acknowledged its responsibility to fund resources for young people and commissioned the Albemarle Report. This was only three months after race riots at Notting Hill and Nottingham, and was clearly a response to the problem of 'dangerous youth', particularly black youth, and male youth. The Youth Service Development Council was set up after the Albemarle Report and largely established the professionally trained and educational youth service of the last three decades. Its perspective in relation to gender was largely on the integration of girls and boys.

The reality behind this official commitment to egalitarianism was that much of the work continued to be with boys alone. Davies, quoting from the National Association of Boys Clubs (1962), asserts that the rationale for this was to allow boys 'to follow male pursuits and to become as good a man as he can possibly be' (1986: 46). Resources for work with girls in single-gender groups, on the other hand, disappeared (Davies 1986). Girls were absorbed into a male-dominated service in which they were marginalised, and they rapidly voted with their feet, using the service much less than boys. Women youth workers also found themselves disadvantaged in a macho world of youth work where the dominant groups, white male youth and white male workers and managers, took control at all levels (Jeffs and Smith 1990; Mansfield 1992).

By the 1970s, feminist workers were demanding girls-only space to compensate for girls' marginalised position in the now pre-dominantly mixed or male-only youth service. In addition, feminists identified the need to develop social education methods which helped young women to understand and challenge the personal and structural effects of sexism. Much literature and a great deal of imaginative and energetic work has gone into establishing girls' work over the past two decades (McRobbie and Nava 1984; Hudson 1987). But this work remains tenuous, as the sudden and peremptory closure of the Girls Work Unit by the National Association of Youth Clubs in 1987 demonstrated (Spence 1990).

PILTON YOUTH PROGRAMME

My work at Pilton Youth Programme mirrors and informs the debates around single-gender work with young people. Pilton Youth Programme (PYP) is a youth project funded jointly by the Education and Social Work Departments of Lothian Regional Council. Its aims are preventive ones: in line with departmental policy, it aims to support young people in trouble at home and in the community, as a preference to residential forms of care. Young people who attend the project come from the Greater Pilton area, a deprived housing scheme on the outskirts of Edinburgh. Some of the highest rates of youth unemployment in Lothian Region are found in Pilton: 28.5 per cent of young men under twenty years, and 22 per cent of all women under twenty years are unemployed (1991 Census Small Area Statistics). Many

families live in sub-standard houses in need of repair and maintenance; others live in high-rise flats.

When PYP opened in 1980, all provision was mixed sex.
Groups referred by social workers, open youth clubs, play-
schemes and counselling took place with little regard to issues of
gender. Like all women youth workers working in a mixed setting,
I found myself operating on an 'if you can't beat them join them'
basis. I learned to play pool and football, and I attempted to
develop my ability to engage in 'banter' in order to survive
alongside male workers, who seemed to command the respect of
young men with ease by using these skills. Hudson is highly
critical of the 'masculinist' ethos which pervades youth work. She
writes: 'In order to work effectively with young and often very
traditionally masculine delinquents, workers need to be assertive,
be able to engage in "bantering" modes of communication, and
also be confident about setting clear boundaries and controls'
(Hudson 1988: 43).

There were undoubtedly losses for the young men as well as
for me in this type-casting of behaviour. The young men greatly
appreciated my ability to empathise and relate warmly to them,
either when they were in small groups or when they were on
their own. But it was impossible for me to respond to them on a
feelings level in a larger group, because the culture of the group
meant that this would have left them feeling vulnerable and
exposed.

In 1989 girls-only groups, run by female staff members, began
for the first time. This was because of a recognition that girls were
regularly outnumbered, marginalised and at times dominated by
boys in the mixed setting. It was also out of an awareness that
girls had different needs from boys. Girls were much less likely
to be referred to PYP because of an offence, unlike boys, and
were much more likely to have come to the notice of a teacher,
parent or social worker because of 'inappropriate behaviour' –
staying out late, sexual activity or choice of friends. Similar
behaviour would probably have been ignored in a boy. Girls'
groups allowed girls and women to talk about growing up to be
women in a sexist society. It also gave girls a safe place to try
out ideas and behaviour and gain confidence, ready to take on
the challenge of a mixed-sex session and a mixed-sex world.

MEN AND BOYS' WORK

Slowly men have been taking up the challenge of boys' work. Stanley (1982) contextualises the entry of radical men, particularly gay men, into work with boys. She argues that a political vacuum caused by disillusionment with socialism and class politics, in addition to the comparative success of feminist thought over the past decade, has given issues of gender a higher profile with the current generation of radical male youth workers, especially gay men (Stanley 1982). The politicising effects of various struggles – the campaign to raise the age of sexual consent for gay men, the crises over AIDS and HIV, and the furore over Clause 28 – have resulted in the emergence of an increasingly strong, organised and confident group of men for whom issues of gender are deeply resonant, but who maintain the power and privileged mantle of their masculinity.

The year 1985 saw the publication of two key texts which illustrate the new concern for gender issues and men in social work/youth work. National Youth Bureau published 'Working with Boys' by Trefor Lloyd and, at the same time, 'Changing the Nature of Masculinity', by Ric Bowl appeared. Since then a gradually growing, although still small boys' work practice has developed, sometimes referred to as 'boyswork'.

Much is currently being made of 'the problem' of masculinity. Feminism has gradually forced an examination of masculinity which has affected men in a variety of ways. Some men have resolved to become less oppressive of women and to work with women against sexism (Hearn and Morgan 1990; Morgan 1992; Seidler 1989). Other men have adopted the language of the women's movement, and use it to describe themselves as victims of their gender and in need of liberation (Irvin 1993). An 'essentialist' approach to the 'crisis' has been propounded by Bly in *Iron John* (Bly 1991) which presents a basic archetypal masculinity from selected ancient myths.

Boys' work is inevitably connected to some of these strands of thought and in particular, the theme of 'father hunger' and the need for boys to find male role models are emphasised by many male youth workers. The argument is that fathers are frequently physically or at least emotionally absent from their children, and so boys have little conception of what an adult male should be like other than through television stereotypes or older boys in the street. Boys are therefore left to piece together an identity from these fragmentary, often violent and aggressive clues (McArthur and Eisen 1976a, 1976b).

In addition, psychological literature suggests that maleness or masculinity is defined negatively – it is formed on the basis of what it is not – and it is not female (Brannon and David 1976; Segal 1990a). This strong desire not to be feminine, fuelled by the low status of women and by homophobia, leads young men to over-compensate and to act out this maleness in an even more exaggerated fashion. Male youth workers, it is argued, can offer boys an example of maleness which is non-aggressive and nurturing and which shows an awareness of feelings. This, of course, is dependent on the male youth worker having these characteristics himself.

PYP began its first all-male boys' group in 1993. The focus of the work with boys since then has been not on their offending behaviour, but instead on the boys' experience of being young and male. An explanation for this can be found in the belief that for the most part, when boys are being 'difficult', they are acting out emotions which they cannot express in other ways because their conditioning as males forbids them. Boys are divided into small groups and are encouraged through activities and discussion to show one another emotional support without the pressure of having to perform in a mixed setting. Residential trips to bothies are valued as a good way of accelerating relationships and assessing individual boys.

Some of the arguments for single-sex work with boys are presented by Boyle and Curtis (1994) as follows:

• In boys/men only settings we do not slip into the tendency to rely on the women or girls to fulfil the role of carer/nurturer, or other so-called 'feminine roles', but take this on ourselves.
• Boys can explore what is interesting to them without dominating girls in the process.
• Boys can learn to accept and see men as available to them emotionally.
• Boys can explore their sexuality with greater ease in front of other males.
• Boys need to be able to express their feelings to men without fear of ridicule or rejection.

- Boys have a desire – however deeply buried – to achieve emotional intimacy with men and with each other.
- If these needs for emotional closeness with men are denied, how then can/do boys express them?

AN ALTERNATIVE APPROACH: ANTI-SEXIST WORK WITH BOYS

As I have described, for political and personal reasons, the move into girls' work meant for many of us feminists working in youth work a move away from work with boys. Difficulties experienced in working with boys in a youth-work setting and, more importantly, the urgent need to establish a service for girls, led feminists to express the view that it was up to male youth workers to 'do something about boys'. I now believe that this is not a satisfactory situation, and that women must reassert their place in working with boys.

Most of the young men who are referred to PYP regularly commit offences such as vandalism, breaking into cars, theft of cars or bikes, and sometimes more violent offences. They are generally young men who are failing in the school system, who have little hope of employment other than very low-paid, casual work. They are the youth of de-industrialised, post-Thatcher Britain. Almost everything in their experience will have told them that they should be strong, powerful, dominant, potent and preferably in possession of a great many consumer goods. Enormous confusion and contradictions are inherent in this situation. As Phillips points out, 'In the barren estates of de-industrialised Britain few men have power for anything other than destruction' (1993: 98). A glance around any barren, peripheral estate bears witness to the reality that this power to destroy is relentlessly used, giving an already bleak environment a threatening and wartorn atmosphere, where people dare not leave their homes empty for fear of break-ins by young male members of their own community (Campbell 1993). Young men exercise their power and experience themselves as powerful in relation to their own small world. Kaufman indicates that some men themselves are victims of social oppression and that a man may 'wield tremendous power in their own milieu and neighbourhood vis-à-vis women of his own class or social groupings or other males' (1994: 152).

One of my major concerns in current boys' work practice is

the non-political nature of this work. The gross reality of gender relations is that men continue to exercise power over women and children in almost every sphere of life. The young men with whom we work are unlikely to have ever considered the possibility of a world which is not structured in this way. Surely the first stage in bringing about change must be to help boys gain an understanding that alternatives are possible and may be desirable? The cost of being the dominant gender is undoubtedly high. Men are more likely to be put in prison, to be murdered, to be homeless, to commit suicide, to be alcoholic, to fail in the education system, to die young, to have fatal accidents – the list goes on (Phillips 1993). Obviously the *status quo*, whilst maintaining men in positions of privilege, results at the same time in many others experiencing great pain and alienation. This pain is where the impetus for change must lie, just as the pain of oppression has led women to bring about change in their lives.

The current tendency of male youth workers involved in this work is to take the position that they are not engaged in anti-sexist work as such, but they are showing boys that there are rewards for achieving greater intimacy with other men and for learning to share and communicate feelings with one another. I believe that in terms of educating young men to find better ways of operating in a world made up of women and men this is not adequate. Bradshaw quotes Grimstead and Rennie (1977) on this point: 'however desirable the reduction of machismo may be for the enrichment of the individual male personality, it has nothing to do with women's freedom' (1982: 184). If we feminists leave this work to men we leave them to deal with 'the inherent contradictions of men trying to organise against their own power' (Bradshaw 1982: 175). Without a woman's perspective, it is too easy for men to forget they have this power.

Men are not, of course, themselves a homogeneous group, so that poor, working-class men and boys are likely to experience oppression themselves to a degree. This is undoubtedly particularly relevant for young black men, who are more likely to be targeted by social control agencies such as police and social work (Hudson 1988). But this reality does not in any way mean that work on power and oppression is not necessary. On the contrary, young working-class men may be encouraged to examine their own contradictory experiences, as they are both powerful and powerless. A boy's work practice which does not in some way attempt to raise awareness of these issues of power, or which on the contrary describes men and boys only in terms of powerlessness, is inadequate. As feminists have developed a girls' work practice which raises awareness of the political issues in relation to sexism and links them to the personal and internal, so boys' awareness might be raised so that they too can link their external experience to their emotional lives.

This takes me to my second area of concern, that men working with boys are not sufficiently motivated to examine and challenge the larger questions in relation to masculinity. The socialisation of boys has for centuries encouraged daring and independence, risk-taking and wild behaviour. This is true regardless of class, but in the case of working class young men it is more likely to take place in public and lead to police action and media vilification. The current boys' work practice is avoiding this global discussion of masculinity in favour of a more personal and introspective model. The argument is that an anti-sexist approach will be too overtly critical of young men's behaviour and may be a 'turn off' for boys (Lloyd 1990).

Patriarchal society has created this risk-taking, independent masculinity for its own self-perpetuation. Feminism has made only a fractional impact on this construction of maleness, and among working-class young men with low levels of literacy, even less than among middle-class men. There seems to me to be a certain naivety in male workers seeing themselves as free enough from their own socialisation to counter the many-layered emotional, intellectual and political foundations of our culture as it is expressed through the behaviour of young men.

I think there is a useful analogy to be made here in connection with issues of race. If white workers declared that they needed an all-white setting in which to work with a group of white young people we might (with some justification) be puzzled and suspicious. If they went on to say that institutional racism was not going to be discussed in case the young people were paralysed by guilt, we would feel even greater scepticism. If they further argued that whites had been hurt just as much as blacks by institutional racism, and that the emphasis of the work was to heal this pain rather than to change the *status quo*, then we really might start to wonder what was going on.

Work with boys places great emphasis on the notion of role models, and this is my third area of anxiety. Lack of male role models is frequently presented as a monolithic explanation for all the destructive and exploitative elements in masculinity. Campbell (1993) offers a rather different perspective on this issue. She argues: 'The lads' problems were not that they were starved of male role models, it was that they were saturated with them' (1993: 323). I would like to suggest that women can provide as good and at times better role models for boys to follow. If women are more able to communicate and co-operate and less likely to commit crimes (Gilligan 1982), why not provide boys with female role models? The answer is that the boys' contempt for women is the problem, rather than their lack of male role models. And this is a problem which can only be addressed by women.

Because men have often partially shut down emotionally themselves, they are not ideally suited to the task of helping young men learn to value characteristics associated with femininity: co-operation and caring (Silverstein and Rashbaun 1994). Our expertise as women is needed to inform this task. It is too important to be left to the men.

There is of course the inevitable question of resources. Already every part of the youth service and the juvenile justice system is dominated by young men. In addition, boys get more use out of recreational facilities in the youth service (Davies 1986). Women workers may feel that any surplus energy they may have is better used to fight the uphill battle of directing resources towards young women. If boys' work is to develop we must ensure that it is not at the expense of already scarce services for young women. However, without a feminist perspective, boys' work is bound to neglect issues which are pressing to women but perhaps of only theoretical interest to male workers. Boys must be enabled to build good, constructive relationships with women, just as they are now able to build different kinds of relationships with men in projects which are run exclusively by men.

CONCLUSION

I do not wish to undermine genuine efforts by men to deal with gender issues in their work with boys. Neither would I wish to blame working-class young men and boys who themselves may experience oppression based on class, youth or race for the sins of men generally. Working-class male teenagers inhabit a hostile world. Society displays a blaming and punitive attitude towards them, enthusiastically inflamed by the popular press. Much is made of their violence and amorality. Why should they behave otherwise in a world where violence is often seen as the officially sanctioned way of dealing with conflict? Their main source of information about the outside world is the popular press, television and films which abound with images of violence both real and fictional.

Meeting these brutalised young men with kindness and understanding, in my experience, often surprises them and brings down some of their barriers. One senses in working with boys how lonely they are, devoid of human contact. Their mothers may have encouraged this distancing, fearing that their influence would leave their sons soft and vulnerable (Silverstein and Rashbaun 1994). Boys often seem to appreciate the chance to experience a relationship with a woman which has some of this warmth and no sexual threat or challenge. It may also give them a different and new idea of what femininity may be.

I believe that by extending humanity to young men and women and by taking them seriously, as male and female workers, we can begin to gain their trust. Once we have earned this trust, they may become interested in our views about the limits of gender, and the ways in which we diminish our lives unnecessarily to fit within these limits. For some young people these ideas may open new possibilities; for others, the alternative ways of seeing may be registered sufficiently to appear in the future when they are needed. Many young men will fail to hear what can only be a whisper when compared with the clamour proclaiming the glory of masculine power reinforced by relentless images of masculinity thrust at them from the screen and in the tabloids.

I have argued that the roots of men's oppressive behaviour are woven into the texture of our culture. As workers with young people, feminists have a potential contribution to make towards unravelling the weave so that both boys and girls can open up to more choices, can be more fully human. The task is an urgent one.

Chapter 11

Moving on

Kate Cavanagh and Viviene E. Cree

In this concluding chapter we will consolidate some of the thinking and ideas which have emerged from this collection with a view to identifying avenues for the further development of feminist theory and practice in social work. We will also present a 'Code of Practice' for work with men, drawing from the range of themes identified by the contributors to this volume.

The central belief shared by all feminists is 'the presupposition that women are oppressed' (Stanley and Wise 1993: 62). For the last two decades, feminist activists, practitioners and academics have expended much energy, in the face of powerful opposition and resistance, to identify the ways in which unequal social divisions between men and women are produced and reproduced. There has been a growing awareness in social work of discrimination against women, both professionally and organisationally (Brook and Davis 1985; Howe 1986) and this has produced strategies for change. This has involved not only the development of women-centred projects and services but also a greater recognition throughout the profession of the need to work collaboratively with women in order to improve their quality of life.

Some assert that feminist practice has made a significant contribution to social work (Dominelli and McLeod 1989). Others are more circumspect (Wise 1990). Mary Langan states of the position of women and social work in the nineties: 'These are difficult times for women and difficult times for social work. Many of the gains of the women's movement over the past twenty years now seem threatened' (1993: 1). We recognise the difficulties of developing and creating feminist practice in a political climate in which the boundaries of welfare provision are being steadily eroded and where social work's focus on anti-discriminatory practice is under threat. Nevertheless, we believe that feminist practitioners remain one of the energising forces in a profession increasingly competence-driven and dominated by management and market ideologies.

One of the fundamental principles underlying the women's movement is a commitment to change: feminism has undoubtedly been influential in changing the lives of women. As women's lives have changed, so have the lives of men. Of greater significance have been the social, political and economic changes which have affected the lives of both men and women. Higher female employment has been accompanied by higher male unemployment. Men of necessity are more involved in household and domestic work; they are more likely to be present at the birth of their babies and to participate in childcare activities (Central Statistics Office 1994).

Despite these changes, men continue to inhabit a privileged position in relation to women. This is undeniable, irrespective of their race or class. Some men have acknowledged that women continue to be discriminated against at all levels of society and have attempted to counter this both personally and professionally. Some have been involved in working collaboratively with women to develop anti-discriminatory strategies, whilst others have concentrated their energies on developing 'men only' services. We believe that whilst 'men only' activities can be influential in encouraging men to explore their masculinities, women and women's experiences *must* inform and influence this work. Segal warns that men working with men may be doing little more than promoting 'new ways to preserve old privileges' (1990a: 281).

We have argued that work with men must be informed by women and women's experiences. Feminist social work must go further than this, however, by making efforts to challenge and change men. This can only be achieved by critically engaging with men and developing a range of strategies which incorporate direct work with men. This may seem contentious given feminism's commitment to forefronting women. However, we believe that women's oppression will not be changed by focusing on women alone and that work with men is therefore a legitimate feminist activity.

This is not without its difficulties. In undertaking work with men, we have experienced many personal and professional dilemmas which we have struggled to resolve. The absence of a feminist literature and practice which might inform our work inevitably compounded an uneasiness born out of attempting to target men. This has increased our resolve to redress this imbalance and to ensure that women undertaking this work are not marginalised.

Bob Connell has asserted that 'men's settled ways of thinking have to be disrupted' (Connell 1989: xii). We feel comfortable with the idea of unsettling men. There is something refreshingly satisfying about the possibility that feminists everywhere in social work *are* busy unsettling, challenging and disturbing men. Writing about our work with men has profoundly affected our consciousness. It has forced an examination of our practice, and this in turn has enabled us to reconsider and reflect on what we have been doing and why we have done it. Our ways of seeing have changed in this process and our feminist lens is stronger.

Specific themes have emerged in our examination of our work with men which we have consolidated in a Code of Practice for Feminist Work with Men.

A CODE OF PRACTICE FOR FEMINIST WORK WITH MEN

Forefronting women – principles

1 Remember that women are our first priority and that work with men is done in order to improve the quality of life for women. It is about recognising that unless men change, then the lives of women and children will not change for the better.
2 Remember that many women *want* men to change. Consider, however, the impact your intervention will have on women with whom those men are in contact.
3 Recognise the pervasiveness of sexual stereotyping and discrimination against women at individual, organisational and societal levels.
4 Acknowledge that work with men is demanding and that support from other women is essential. Value other women who are doing this work. Networks are important.
5 Identify the ways in which your own values and experiences influence your work with men and women.

Forefronting men – principles

1 Remember that work with men is one aspect of a broader feminist strategy for changing unequal power relations between men and women.
2 Be aware of the ways in which men can experience oppression – for example, on the basis of class, race, sexual orientation. Link the commonalities.
3 Be open to the reality that some men want to change and men have much to gain from change.
4 Remember that services for men should not detract from services to women.
5 Men can only know how women experience oppression from women themselves.

Change

1 Acknowledge that change is a central objective of the feminist agenda and that both women and men are an integral part of the change process.
2 Remember that change has a political component as well as a personal component and that change must take place at both levels.
3 Remember that change is possible but change can be difficult – it can involve giving something up and it is often accompanied by resistance, bitterness and anger. Change is a process and is seldom immediate.
4 Identify the best possible strategies for implementing change and review your progress regularly. Evaluating effectiveness is essential in developing and promoting creative and productive practices.

Strategies

1 Planning and preparation

Preparation is essential. Identify your objectives, how you plan to proceed and what supports are available to you. Anticipate resistance and be aware of the diverse ways in which resistance can be expressed – for example, anger, defensiveness, excuses, minimisation. Know the feminist theoretical framework within which you are operating. Rehearse the arguments and practise techniques so that you are confident of your knowledge, value-base and skills.

2 Roles

Resist the temptation to conform to men's stereotypical expectations of women – for example, mother, comforter, partner, shoulder to cry on. Consider ways of interacting with men which challenge stereotypical role expectations and be aware of the pressures to collude and to compromise.

3 Challenge

Challenges must be constructive and effective. Avoid outright confrontation or conflict, which is often counter-productive. Scapegoating and stereotyping may produce guilt and defensiveness. Remember that men are not accustomed to being challenged by women; anticipate possible reactions, including anger, denial, blaming. Do not expect to challenge every expression of sexism. Conserve your energies for those on whom you think you can have an impact. Timing is important. Choose when, where, why, how and in what way to challenge.

4 Critical engagement

Be aware that it is important to listen to men. Be open to hearing about their experiences and views but do so with a strong feminist lens. Be prepared to engage with men with an open mind and a feminist perspective. Recognise the difficulties some men have in expressing feelings.

5 Power and control

Maintain your own integrity in the face of men's efforts to exert power and control. Consider how you might best achieve this – for example, assertiveness training, rehearsing arguments, role-playing and co-working may all be useful. Be aware that men may attempt to divest you of professional and personal power.

6 Methods of working with men

It may be useful to draw on strategies from the women's movement, including consciousness-raising, group work, examination of the social construction of gender. But more fundamental than this, we must acknowledge that personal matters are also political issues. It is *feminist* practice which is our goal. Gender-sensitive practice and gender equality practice are not enough.

> If women's lives cannot be liberated without the simultaneous transformation of gendered production systems, then men cannot sensibly be left out of women's struggles. This does not mean that women who want to lead separate lives should have to work with men. The contradictions of feminist theory show quite clearly the need to struggle with men while simultaneously struggling against them.
>
> (Ramazonoğlu 1989: 189–90)

Bibliography

Abbott, P. and Wallace, C. (1990) *An Introduction to Sociology: Feminist Perspectives*, London: Routledge.

Abramovitz, M. (1985) 'Status of women on faculty and status of women's studies in Israeli schools of social work', *Social Work Education* 4(3): 3–6.

—— (1987) 'Making gender a variable in social work teaching', *Journal of Teaching in Social Work* 1: 29–52.

Adams, D. (1988) 'Treatment models of men who batter: a profeminist analysis', in K. Yllo and M. L. Bograd (eds) *Feminist Perspectives on Wife Abuse*, Newbury Park, Cal.: Sage.

Afshar, H. and Maynard, M. (1994) *The Dynamics of 'Race' and Gender: Some Feminist Interventions*, London: Taylor and Francis.

Alcoff, L. and Potter, E. (1993) *Feminist Epistemologies*, New York: Routledge.

Allen, G. (1992) 'Active citizenship: a rationale for the education of citizens?', in G. Allen and I. Martin (eds) *Education and Community: The Politics of Practice*, London: Cassell.

Allen, G., Bastiani, I. and Richard, K. (eds) (1987) *Community Education: An Agenda for Educational Reform*, Milton Keynes: Open University Press.

Ambrose, P., Harper, J. and Pemberton, R. (1983) *Surviving Divorce: Men beyond Marriage*, Brighton: Wheatsheaf.

Anthias, F. and Yuval-Davis, N. (1983) 'Contextualising feminism: gender, ethnic and class divisions', *Feminist Review* 15: 62–75.

Arber, S. and Gilbert, N. (1989) 'Men: the forgotten carers', *Sociology* 23(1): 111–18.

Archer, J. (1989) 'The relationship between gender-role measures: a review', *British Journal of Social Psychology* 28(2): 173–84.

Archer, J. and Lloyd, B. B. (1985) *Sex and Gender*, Cambridge: Cambridge University Press.

Bailey, R. and Brake, M. (eds) (1980) *Radical Social Work and Practices*, London: Edward Arnold.

Bailey, S. and Cox, P. (1993) 'Teaching gender issues on social work courses', *Social Work Education* 12(1): 19–35.

Baker Miller, J. (1978) *Towards a New Psychology for Women*, London: Pelican.

Bancroft, J. (1989) *Human Sexuality and its Problems*, 2nd edn, Edinburgh: Churchill Livingstone.

Barrett, M. (1980) *Women's Oppression Today: The Marxist-Feminist Encounter*, London: Verso.

Barrett, M. and McIntosh, M. (1982) *The Anti-Social Family* London: Verso.

Barrett, M. and Phillips, A. (1992) *Destabilizing Theory: Contemporary Feminist Debates*, Cambridge: Polity Press.

Bart, P. B. and Moran, E. G. (eds) (1993) *Violence against Women: The Bloody Footprints*, Newbury Park, Cal.: Sage.

Beagley, J. (1986) 'Why men manage and women are the workforce', *Community Care* (Supplement), 18 Sept.

Bell, C. and Roberts, H. (eds) (1984) *Social Researching: Politics, Problems, Practice*, London: Routledge.

Bem, S. L. (1974) 'The measurement of psychological androgyny', *Journal of Consulting and Clinical Psychology* 42(2): 155–62.

—— (1977) 'On the utility of alternate procedures for assessing psychological androgyny', *Journal of Consulting and Clinical Psychology* 45: 196–205.

Bertaux, D. (ed.) (1981) *Biography and Society*, Newbury Park, Cal.: Sage.

Bhavnani, K. and Coulson, M. (1986) 'Transforming socialist-feminism: the challenge of racism', *Feminist Review* 23.

Bly, R. (1991) *Iron John: A Book about Men*, Shaftesbury: Element.

Bograd, M. L. (1988) 'Feminist perspectives on wife abuse: an introduction', in K. Yllo and M. L. Bograd (eds) *Feminist Perspectives on Wife Abuse*, Newbury Park, Cal.: Sage.

Boreham, N. C. and Arthur, T. A. A. (1993) *Information Requirements and Occupational Decision Making*, London: Department of Employment.

Boston Women's Health Collective (1976) *Our Bodies Our Selves: A Health Book by, and for, Women*, New York: Simon and Schuster.

Bourne, J. (1983) 'Towards an anti racist feminism', *Race and Class* 25 (1).

Boushel, M. (1991) 'Anti-discriminatory work in placement: helping students prepare', *Social Work Education* 10(3): 51–69.

Bowl, R. (1985) *Changing the Nature of Masculinity: A Task for Social Work*, Norwich, University of East Anglia in association with *Social Work Today*.

Bowles, G. and Duelli Klein, R. (eds) (1983) *Theories of Women's Studies*, London: Routledge and Kegan Paul.

Boyle, R. and Curtis, K. (1994) *Breaking the Chain*, Edinburgh: Pilton Youth Programme.

Bradshaw, J. (1982) 'Now what are they up to? Men in the "men's movement"!', in S. Friedman and E. Sarah (eds) *On the Problem of Men: Two Feminist Conferences*, London: Women's Press.

Brady, P. (1989) 'Towards anti-sexist practice', in R. Canton (ed.) *Learn-*

ing at Work: Essays by Teachers of Social Work Practice, London: Central Council for Education and Training in Social Work.

Brannen, J. (ed.) (1992) *Mixing Methods: Qualitative and Quantitative Research*, Aldershot: Avebury.

Brannon, R. and David, D. S. (1976) 'The male sex role: our culture's blueprint of manhood, and what it's done for us lately', in D. S. David and R. Brannon (eds) *The Forty-nine Per Cent Majority*, Reading, Mass.: Addison-Wesley.

Brittan, A. (1989) *Masculinity and Power*, Oxford: Blackwell.

Brod, H. (ed.) (1987) *The Making of Masculinities: The New Men's Studies*, Boston, Mass.: Allen and Unwin.

Brod, H. and Kaufman, M. (eds) (1994) *Theorising Masculinities*, London: Sage.

Brook, E. and Davis, A. (eds) (1985) *Women: The Family and Social Work*, London: Tavistock.

Brown, W. (1983) *Black Women and the Peace Movement*, Bristol: Falling Wall Press.

Brownmiller, S. (1986) *Femininity*, London: Paladin.

Bryman, A. (1988) *Quantity and Quality in Social Research*, London: Unwin Hyman.

Burns, J. and Wright, C. (1993) *Sexuality in the Context of HIV/AIDS: A Guide to Workshops for People who Work with Young People*, London: HMSO.

Burns, N., Meredith, C. and Paquetti, C. (1991) *Treatment Programs for Men who Batter: A Review of the Evidence of their Success*, Ontario: Abt Associates of Canada.

Cain, M. (1986) 'Realist philosophy and standpoint epistemologies or feminist criminology as a successor science', in L. Gelsthorpe and A. Morris (eds) *Feminist Perspectives in Criminology*, Milton Keynes: Open University.

—— (ed.) (1989) *Growing Up Good: Policing the Behaviour of Girls in Europe*, London: Sage.

Campbell, B. (1993) *Goliath: Britain's Dangerous Places*, London: Methuen.

Campbell, J. (1994) 'The great divide of race', *The Scotsman*, 3 Dec.

Canaan, J. E. and Griffin, C. (1990) 'The new men's studies: part of the problem or part of the solution?', in J. Hearn and D. H. J. Morgan (eds) *Men, Masculinities and Social Theory*, London: Open University.

Canton, R. (ed.) (1989) *Learning at Work: Essays by Teachers of Social Work Practice*, London: Central Council for Education and Training in Social Work.

Caplan, P. J. (1993) *Lifting a Ton of Feathers: A Woman's Guide to Surviving in the Academic World*, Toronto: University of Toronto Press.

Carby, H. V. (1982) 'White woman listen: black feminism and the boundaries of sisterhood', in *The Empire Strikes Back: Race and Racism in 70s Britain*, London: Hutchinson and Centre for Contemporary Cultural Studies.

Carlen, P. (1983) *Women's Imprisonment*, London: Routledge.

—— (1988) *Women, Crime and Poverty*, Milton Keynes: Open University Press.

Carli, L. (1990) 'Gender, language and influence', *Journal of Personality and Social Psychology* 59(5): 941–51.

Carlson, N. L. (1987) 'Women therapist: male client', in M. Scher, M. Stevens, G. Good and G. A. Eichenfield (eds) *Handbook of Counseling and Psychotherapy with Men*, Newbury Park, Cal.: Sage.

Carter, P., Everitt, A. and Hudson, A. (1992) 'Malestream training? Women, feminism and social work education', in M. Langan and L. Day (eds) *Women, Oppression and Social Work: Issues in Anti-discriminatory Practice*, London: Routledge.

Central Council for Education and Training in Social Work (1989) *Requirements and Regulations for the Diploma in Social Work DipSW*, London: CCETSW.

Central Statistical Office (1994) *Social Trends*, London: HMSO.

Centre for Contemporary Cultural Studies (1982) *The Empire Strikes Back: Race and Racism in 70s Britain*, London: Hutchinson and Centre for Contemporary Cultural Studies.

Chafetz, J. S. (1972) 'Women in social work', *Social Work* 17(5) (Sept.).

Chaplin, J. (1988) *Feminist Counselling in Action*, London: Sage.

Chapman, R. and Rutherford, J. (1988) *Male Order: Unwrapping Masculinity*, London: Lawrence and Wishart.

Chodorow, N. (1978) *The Reproduction of Mothering: Psychoanalysis and the Sociology of Gender*, Berkeley, Cal.: University of California Press.

—— (1980) 'Gender relation and difference in psychoanalytic perspectives', in H. Eisenstein and A. Jardine (eds) *The Future of Difference*, New Brunswick, NJ.: Rutgers University Press.

Chusmir, L. C. (1983) 'Characteristics and predictive dimensions of women who make nontraditional vocational choices', *The Personnel and Guidance Journal* 62(1): 43–7.

—— (1990) 'Men who make nontraditional career choices', *Journal of Counseling and Development* 69: 11–16.

Cockburn, C. (1991) *In the Way of Women: Men's Resistance to Sex Equality in Organizations*, Basingstoke: Macmillan.

Connell, R. W. (1987) *Gender and Power: Society, the Person and Sexual Politics*, Oxford: Blackwell.

—— (1989) 'Cool guys, wimps and swots: the interplay of masculinity and education', *Oxford Review of Education* 15 (3).

—— (1993) 'Drumming up the wrong tree', *Tikkun* 7(1).

Cook, J. and Fonow, M. (1986) 'Knowledge and women's interests: issues of epistemology and methodology in feminist social research', *Sociological Inquiry* 56: 2–29.

Coyle, A. (1991) *Inside: Rethinking Scotland's Prisons*, Edinburgh: Scottish Child.

Crawley, J. (1983) 'Experiential methods in social work education', *Social Work Education*, 3(1).

Cree, V. E. (1995) *From Public Streets to Private Lives: The Changing Task of Social Work*, Aldershot: Avebury.

Crompton, R. and Sanderson, K. (1990) *Gendered Jobs and Social Change*, London: Unwin Hyman.

Dale, J. and Foster, P. (1986) *Feminists and State Welfare*, London: Routledge & Kegan Paul.

David, D. S. and Brannon, R. (eds) (1987) *The Forty-nine Per Cent Majority*, Reading, Mass.: Addison-Wesley.

Davies, B. (1986) *Threatening Youth Towards a National Youth Policy*, Milton Keynes: Open University Press.

Davis, A. (1981) *Women, Race and Class*, London: Women's Press.

Denzin, N. K. (1970). *The Research Act in Sociology: A Theoretical Introduction to Sociological Methods*, London: Butterworths.

Dobash, R. E. and Dobash, R. P. (1979) *Violence against Wives: A Case against the Patriarchy*, New York: Free Press.

—— (1981) 'Social sciences and social action: the case of wife beating', *Journal of Family Issues* 2(4): 439–70.

—— (1988) 'Research as social action: the struggle for battered women, in K. Yllo and M. Bograd (eds) *Feminist Perspectives on Wife Abuse* Newbury Park, Cal.: Sage.

—— (1992) *Women, Violence and Social Change*, London: Routledge.

Dobash, R. E., Dobash, R. P., Cavanagh, K. and Lewis, R. (1995a) 'Evaluating British and American approaches to domestic violence interventions', in R. P. Dobash, R. E. Dobash and L. Noaks (eds) *Crime and Gender*, Cardiff: University of Wales Press.

—— (1995b) *Research Evaluation of Programmes for Violent Men*. Ediburgh: Scottish Office (in publication).

Dobash, R. P., Carnie, J. and Waterhouse, L. (1993) 'Child sexual abusers: recognition and response', in L. Waterhouse (ed.) *Child Abuse and Child Abusers: Protection and Prevention*, London: Kingsley.

Dobash, R. P. and Dobash, R. E. (1981) 'Community responses to violence against wives: abstract justice and patriarchy', *Social Problems* 28(5).

—— (1983) 'The context-specific approach', in D. Finkelhor, G. Hotaling, R. Gelles and M. Straus (eds) *The Dark Side of Families: Current Family Violence Research*, Newbury Park, Cal.: Sage.

Dobash, R. P., Dobash, R. E. and Noaks, L. (eds) (1995) *Gender and Crime*, Cardiff: University of Wales Press.

Dominelli, L. and McLeod, E. (1989) *Feminist Social Work*, Basingstoke: Macmillan.

Du Bois, B. (1983) 'Passionate scholarship: notes on values, knowing and methods in feminist social science', in G. Bowles and R. Duelli Klein (eds) *Theories of Women's Studies*, London: Routledge and Kegan Paul.

Duff, A., Dobash, R. E., Marshall, S. and Dobash, R. P. (eds) (1994) *Penal Theory and Practice: Tradition and Innovation in Criminal Justice*, Manchester: Manchester University Press.

Dworkin, A. (1981) *Pornography: Men Possessing Women*, London: Women's Press.

—— (1988) *Letters from a War Zone: Writings 1976–1987*, London: Secker and Warburg.

Eardley, T. (1991) 'Men's work', in V. Seidler (ed.) *The Achilles Heel Reader*, London: Routledge.

Edleson, J. L., Miller, D. and Stone, G. W. (1985) *Counseling Men who Batter: Group Leader's Handbook*, Albany, NY: Men's Coalition Against Battering.

Edleson, J. L. and Syers, M. (1989) *The Relative Effectiveness of Group Treatments for Men who Batter*, Minneapolis, Minn.: Domestic Abuse Project.

Edleson, J. L. and Tolman, R. M. (1992) *Intervention for Men who Batter: An Ecological Approach*, London: Sage.

Edwards, S. (1989) *Policing Domestic Violence – Women, the Law and the State*, London: Sage.

Eichenbaum, L. and Orbach, S. (1985) *Understanding Women*, Harmondsworth: Penguin.

Eisenstein, H. and Jardine, A. (eds) (1980) *The Future of Difference*, New Brunswick, NJ: Rutgers University Press.

Eisikovits, Z. C. and Edleson, J. L. (1989) 'Intervening with men who batter: a critical review of the literature', *Social Service Review* 63(3): 384–414.

Faludi, S. (1992) *Backlash: The Undeclared War against Women*, London: Chatto and Windus.

Faragher, T. (1985) 'The police response to violence against women in the home', in J. Pahl, (ed.) *Private Violence and Public Policy: The Needs of Battered Women and the Response of Public Services*, London: Routledge.

Faulk, R. (1973) 'Men who assault their wives', *Medical Science and the Law* 14: 180–3.

Finch, J. (1984) 'It's great to have someone to talk to: the ethics and politics of interviewing women', in C. Bell and H. Roberts (eds) *Social Researching: Politics, Problems, Practice*, London: Routledge.

—— (1989) *Family Obligations and Social Change*, Cambridge: Polity Press.

Finkelhor, D., Hotaling, G., Gelles, R. and Strause, M. (eds) (1983) *The Dark Side of Families: Current Family Violence Research*, Newbury Park, Cal.: Sage.

Firestone, S. (1979) *The Dialectic of Sex: The Case for Feminist Revolution*, London: Women's Press.

Fonow, M. and Cook, J. (1992) *Beyond Methodology: Feminist Scholarship as Lived Research*, Bloomington, Ind.: Indiana University Press.

Ford, A. (1985) *Men: A Documentary*, London: Weidenfeld and Nicolson.

Formaini, H. (1990) *Men: The Darker Continent*, London: Heinemann.

Forster, J. (1988) 'Divorce advice and counselling for men', Edinburgh: Scottish Marriage Guidance Council.

Foucault, M. (1972) *The Archaeology of Knowledge*, London: Tavistock.

Friedman, S. and Sarah, E. (eds) (1982) *On the Problem of Men: Two Feminist Conferences*, London: Women's Press.

Friere, P. (1972) *The Pedagogy of the Oppressed*, Harmondsworth: Penguin.

Galbraith, M. (1992) 'Understanding career choices of men in elementary education', *Journal of Educational Research* 85(4): 246–53.

Gamarnikow, E. (ed.) (1986) *The Public and the Private*, Papers presented at the 1985 Annual Conference of the British Sociological Association, Aldershot: Gower.

Garland, D. (1985) *Punishment and Welfare*, Aldershot: Gower.

Gayford, J. J. (1975) 'Wife beating: a preliminary survey of 100 cases', *British Medical Journal* 1: 194–7.

Gelles, R. J. (1972) *The Violent Home: A Study of Physical Aggression between Husbands and Wives*, Beverly Hills, Cal.: Sage.

Gelsthorpe, L. (1987) 'The differential treatment of males and females in the criminal justice system', in Research Highlights in Social Work, *Sex, Gender and Care Work*, London: Jessica Kingsley.

Gelsthorpe, L. and Morris, A. (eds) (1986) *Feminist Perspectives in Criminology*, Milton Keynes: Open University.

Gilbert, N. (ed.) (1990) *Researching Social Life*, London: Sage.

Gilligan, C. (1982) *In a Different Voice: Psychological Theory and Women's Development*, Cambridge, Mass.: Harvard University Press.

Giroux, H. A. (1992) *Border Crossings: Cultural Workers and the Politics of Education*, New York: Routledge.

Glendinning, C. and Millar, J. (eds) (1987) *Women and Poverty in Britain*, Brighton: Wheatsheaf.

Golan, N. (1978) *Treatment in Crisis Situations*, New York: Free Press.

Goode, W. J. (1971) 'Force and violence in the family', *Journal of Marriage and the Family* 33(4): 624–36.

Gordon, L. (1991) 'On difference', *Genders* 10 Spring.

Grant, J. (1993) *Fundamental Feminism: Contesting the Core Concepts of Feminist Theory*, London: Routledge.

Great Britain. Home Office (1990) *Criminal Justice and Protecting the Public*, London: HMSO (Cmd 965).

—— Scottish Home and Health Department (1990) *Investigation of Complaints of Domestic Assault* (Police (CC) Circular No 3/1990), Edinburgh: Scottish Home and Health Department.

—— Scottish Office. Social Work Services Group (1991) *National Objectives and Standards for Social Work Services in the Criminal Justice System*, Edinburgh: Social Work Service Group.

Grimstead, K. and Rennie, S. (1977) 'Men', in J. Snodgrass (ed.) *A Book of Readings for Men Against Sexism*, New York: Times Change Press.

Grimwood, C. and Popplestone, R. (eds) (1993) *Women, Management and Care*, Basingstoke: Macmillan.

Hagan, K. (ed.) (1992) *Women Respond to the Men's Movement: A Feminist Collection*, San Francisco, Cal.: Pandora.

Hague, G. and Malos, E. (1993) *Domestic Violence: Action for Change*, Cheltenham: New Clarion Press.

Hale, J. (1984) 'Feminism and social work practice', in B. Jordan and N. Parton (eds) *The Political Dimensions of Social Work*, Oxford: Blackwell.

Hanmer, J. and Maynard, M. (eds) (1987) *Women, Violence and Social Control*, Basingstoke: Macmillan.

Hanmer, J. and Rose, H. (1980) 'Making sense of theory', in P. Henderson, D. Jones and D. N. Thomas (eds) *The Boundaries of Change in
Community Work*, London: Allen and Unwin.

Hanmer, J. and Statham, D. (1988) *Women and Social Work: Towards a
Woman-centred Practice*, London: Macmillan.

Harding, S. (1987) *Feminism and Methodology: Social Science Issues*,
Bloomington, Ind.: Indiana University Press.

Harding, S. (1991) *Whose Science? Whose Knowledge? Thinking from
Women's Lives*, Milton Keynes: Open University Press.

Harper, J. (1987) 'Men as workers and clients', *Community Care (Inside)*,
25 June.

Hart, B. (1988) *Safety for Women: Monitoring Batterers' Programs*,
Harrisburg, Pa.: Pennsylvania Coalition against Domestic Violence.

Hearn, J. (1987) *The Gender of Oppression: Men, Masculinity and the
Critique of Marxism*, Brighton: Wheatsheaf.

Hearn, J. and Morgan, D. H. J. (1990) *Men, Masculinities and Social
Theory*, London: Unwin Hyman.

Hekman, S. (1990) *Gender and Knowledge: Elements of a Postmodern
Feminism*, Cambridge: Polity Press.

Henderson, P., Jones, D. and Thomas, D. N. (eds) (1980) *The Boundaries
of Change in Community Work*, London: Allen and Unwin.

Hetherington, E. M., Cox, M. and Cox, R. (1976) 'Divorced fathers',
The Family Coordinator, Oct.: 417–28.

Hochschild, A. (1990) *The Second Shift: Working Parents and the Revolution*, London: Piatkus.

Hodson, P. (1984) *Men: An Investigation into the Emotional Male*,
London: BBC Books.

Holland, J. and Ramazanoğlu, C. (1994) 'Coming to conclusions: power
and interpretation', in M. Maynard and J. Purvis (eds) *Researching
Women's Lives from a Feminist Perspective*, London: Taylor Francis.

Home Office (1990) *Prison Statistics*, London: HMSO.

hooks, b. (1983) *Ain't I A Woman: Black Women and Feminism*, 2nd
edn, London: Pluto.

—— (1984) *Feminist Theory: From Margin to Centre*, Boston, Mass.:
South End Books.

—— (1989) *Talking Back: Thinking Feminist, Thinking Black*, London:
Sheba Press.

—— (1992) 'Men in feminist struggle: the necessary movement', in K.
Hagan (ed.) *Women Respond to the Men's Movement: A Feminist
Collection*, San Francisco, Cal.: Pandora.

Howe, D. (1986) 'The segregation of women and their work in the
personal social services', *Critical Social Policy* 15: 21–36.

Hoyland, J. (ed.) (1992) *Fathers and Sons*, London: Serpent's Tail.

Hudson, A. (1985) 'Feminism and social work: resistance or dialogue?',
British Journal of Social Work 15 (Dec.).

—— (1987) 'Troublesome girls: towards alternative definitions and policies', in M. Cain (ed.) *Growing up Good: Policing the Behaviour of
Girls in Europe*, London: Sage.

—— (1988) 'Boys will be boys: masculinism and the juvenile justice system', *Critical Social Policy* 21: 30–48.

—— (1989) 'Changing perspectives: feminism, gender and social work', in M. Langan and P. Lee (eds) *Radical Social Work Today*, London: Unwin.

—— (1992) 'The child sexual abuse "industry" and gender relations in social work', in M. Langan and L. Day (eds) *Women, Oppression and Social Work: Issues in Anti-discriminatory Practice*, London: Routledge.

—— (1995) *Troublesome Girls: Adolescence, Femininity and the State*, Basingstoke: Macmillan.

Humphries, B. (1989) 'Adult learning in social work education: towards liberation or domestication?', *Critical Social Policy* 33.

Irvin, J. (1993) *The Liberation of Males*, Washington: Rational Island.

Jacobs, H. (1988) *Incidents in the Life of a Slave Girl*, Oxford: Oxford University Press.

Jacobs, J. A. (1993) 'Men in female-dominated fields: trends and turnover', in C. L. Williams (ed.) *Doing Women's Work: Men in Non-traditional Occupations*, Newbury Park, Cal.: Sage.

Jacobs, J. W. (1982) 'The effect of divorce on fathers: an overview of the literature', *American Journal of Psychiatry* 130(10): 1235–41.

Jardine, A. and Smith, P. (1987) *Men in Feminism*, London: Routledge.

Jeffs, T. and Smith, M. (eds) (1990) *Youth Work and Gender*, London: Macmillan.

Johnson, N. (ed.) (1985a) *Marital Violence (Sociological Review* monograph: 31), London: Routledge.

—— (1985b) 'Police, social work and medical responses to battered women', in N. Johnson (ed.) *Marital Violence (Sociological Review* monograph: 31), London: Routledge.

Jordan, B. and Parton, N. (eds) (1983) *The Political Dimensions of Social Work*, Oxford: Blackwell.

Jordan, P. (1985) *Men Hurt*, Melbourne: Family Court of Australia.

Kadushin, A. (1976) 'Men in a woman's profession', *Social Work* 21(6): 440–7.

Kaufman, M. (1994) 'Men, feminism and men's contradictory experiences of power', in H. Brod and M. Kaufman (eds) *Theorising Masculinities*, London: Sage.

Kearney, P. and Le Riche, P. (1993) 'Looking at the ordinary in a new way: the applications of feminist thinking to a post-qualifying social work course', *Social Work Education* 12(2).

Kelly, L. (1988) *Surviving Sexual Violence*, Cambridge: Polity Press.

Kelly, L., Burton, S. and Regan, L. (1994) 'Researching women's lives or studying women's oppression? Reflections on what constitutes feminist research', in M. Maynard and J. Purvis (eds) *Researching Women's Lives from a Feminist Perspective*, London: Taylor Francis.

Kirk, S. and Rosenblatt, A. (1984) 'The contribution of women faculty members to social work journals', *Social Work* 29(1): 67–9.

Kravetz, D. (1976) 'Sexism in a woman's profession', *Social Work* 21(6): 421–6.

Kruk, E. (1989) 'Impact of divorce on non-custodial fathers', unpublished Ph.D. thesis, University of Edinburgh.

La Valle, I. and Lyons, K. (1993) 'Gender differences in social workers' career paths', *Women's Link* 3: 2.

Lakoff, R. T. (1975) *Language and Woman's Place*, New York: Harper and Row.

Langan, M. (1992) 'Introduction: women and social work in the nineties', in M. Langan and L. Day (eds) *Women, Oppression and Social Work: Issues in Anti-discriminatory Practice*, London: Routledge.

Langan, M. and Day, L. (eds) (1992) *Women, Oppression and Social Work: Issues in Anti-discriminatory Practice*, London: Routledge.

Langan, M. and Lee, P. (eds) (1989) *Radical Social Work Today*, London: Unwin.

Lather, P. A. (1991) *Getting Smart: Feminist Research and Pedagogy with/in the Postmodern World*, New York: Routledge.

Lemkau, J. P. (1984) 'Men in female-dominated professions: distinguishing personality and background features', *Journal of Vocational Behaviour* 24: 110–22.

Lennon, K. and Whitford, M. (1994) *Knowing the Difference: Feminist Perspectives in Epistemology*, London: Routledge.

Levitas, R. (ed.) (1986) *The Ideology of the New Right*, Cambridge: Polity Press.

Lewis, C. and O'Brian, M. (eds) (1987) *Reassessing Fatherhood: New Observations on Fathers and the Modern Family*, London: Sage.

Lloyd, T. (1985) *Working with Boys*, Leicester: National Youth Bureau.

—— (1990) 'Cornerstones of boys' work', *Working with Men*, Oct., 10.

Longino, H. E. (1993) 'Feminist standpoint theory and the problems of knowledge', *Signs* 19(1): 201–12.

Lupton, C. and Gillespie, T. (eds) (1994) *Working with Violence*, Basingstoke: Macmillan.

Lyndon, N. (1992) *No More Sex War: The Failures of Feminism*, London: Sinclair-Stevenson.

McArthur, L. and Eisen, S. (1976a) 'Achievements of male and female story book characters as determinants of achievement behavior by boys and girls', *Journal of Personality and Social Psychology* 33(4): 467–73

—— (1976b) 'Television and sex role stereotyping', *Journal of Applied Social Psychology* 6: 329–51.

McCormack, M. (1990) *Divorce and After: The Father's Tales*, London: Macdonald Optima.

McDowell, L. and Pringle, R. (eds) (1992) *Defining Women: Social Institutions and Gender Divisions*, Cambridge: Polity Press.

McGuire, J. and Priestley, P. (1985) *Offending Behaviour: Skills and Stratagems for Going Straight*, London: Batsford.

McKee, L. and O'Brien, M. (1983) 'Interviewing men: taking gender seriously', in E. Gamarnikow (ed) *The Public and the Private*, London: Heinemann.

McLeod, E. (1987) 'Some lessons from teaching feminist social work', *Issues in Social Work Education* 7(1).

MacLeod, M. and Saraga, E. (1988) 'Challenging the orthodoxy: towards a feminist theory and practice', *Feminist Review* 28: 16–56.

McRobbie, A. and Nava, M. (eds) (1984) *Gender and Generation*, London: Macmillan.

Mansfield, S. (1992) *Education and Community*, London: Cassell.

Marshall, W. L. and Barbaree, H. E. (1990) 'Outcome of comprehensive behavioural treatment programs', in W. L. Marshall, D. R. Laws and H. E. Barbaree (eds) *Handbook of Sexual Assault*, New York: Plenum Press.

Marshall, W. L., Laws, D. R. and Barbaree, H. E. (eds) (1990) *Handbook of Sexual Assault*, New York: Plenum Press.

Martin, I. (1987) 'Community education: towards a theoretical analysis', in G. Allen, J. Bastiani, I. Martin and K. Richards (eds) *Community Education: An Agenda for Educational Reform*, Milton Keynes: Open University.

May, T. (1993) *Social Research: Issues, Methods, and Process*, Buckingham: Open University Press.

Maynard, M. (1990) 'The re-shaping of sociology? Trends in the study of gender', *Sociology* 24(2): 269–90.

—— (1994) 'Methods, practice and epistemology: the debate about feminism and research', in M. Maynard and J. Purvis (eds) *Researching Women's Lives from a Feminist Perspective*, London: Taylor and Francis.

Maynard, M. and Purvis, J. (eds) (1994) *Researching Women's Lives from a Feminist Perspective*, London: Taylor Francis.

Mies, M. (1983) 'Towards a methodology for feminist research', in G. Bowles and R. Duelli-Klein (eds) *Theories of Women's Studies*, London: Routledge and Kegan Paul.

Mitchell, J. and Oakley, A. (eds) (1986) *What is Feminism?* Oxford: Blackwell.

Mitter, S. (1986) *Common Fate, Common Bond: Women in the Global Economy*, London: Pluto.

Moore, G. and Wood, C. (1992) *Moore and Wood's Social Work and Criminal Law in Scotland*, 2nd edn, Edinburgh: Mercat Press.

Moraga, C. and Anzaldua, G. (eds) (1981) *This Bridge Called My Back: Writings by Radical Women of Color*, Watertown, Mass.: Persephone Press.

Morgan, D. H. J. (1992) *Discovering Men*, London: Routledge.

Morran, D. and Wilson, M. (1994) 'Confronting domestic violence: an innovative criminal justice response in Scotland', in A. Duff *et al.* (eds) *Penal Theory and Practice: Tradition and Innovation in Criminal Justice*, Manchester: Manchester University Press.

Neustatter, A. (1994) *Guardian*, 2 September.

Newton, C. (1994) 'Gender theory and prison sociology: using theories of masculinities to interpret the sociology of prisons for men', *The Howard Journal* 33(3).

Oakley, A. (1981) 'Interviewing women: a contradiction in terms', in H. Roberts (ed.) *Doing Feminist Research*, London: Routledge and Kegan Paul.

—— (1985) *Subject Women*, London: Fontana.
Pahl, J. (ed.) (1985) *Private Violence and Public Policy: The Needs of Battered Women and the Response of Public Services*, London: Routledge and Kegan Paul.
Pascall, G. (1986) *Social Policy: A Feminist Analysis*, London: Tavistock.
Pateman, C. (1987) 'Feminist critiques of the public–private dichotomy', in A. Phillips (ed.) *Feminism and Equality*, Oxford: Blackwell.
Pearson, G. (1983) *Hooligan: A History of Respectable Fears*, London: Macmillan.
Pence, E. and Paymar, M. (1990) *Power and Control: Tactics of Men who Batter*, Duluth, Minn.: Minnesota Program Development.
Pence, E. and Shepard, M. (1988) 'Integrating feminist theory and practice: the challenge of the battered women's movement', in K. Yllo and M. L. Bograd (eds) *Feminist Perspectives on Wife Abuse*, Newbury Park, Cal.: Sage.
Perrott, S. (1994) 'Working with men who abuse men and children', in C. Lupton and T. Gillespie (eds) *Working with Violence*, Basingstoke: Macmillan.
Phillips, A. (ed.) (1987) *Feminism and Equality*, Oxford: Blackwell.
—— (1993) *The Trouble with Boys*, London: Pandora.
Phillipson, J. (1992) *Practising Equality: Women, Men and Social Work*, London: Central Council for Education and Training in Social Work.
—— (1993) 'Managing with style', in C. Grimwood and R. Popplestone (eds) *Women, Management and Care*, Basingstoke: Macmillan.
Pirog-Good, M. and Stets-Kealy, J. (1985) 'Male batterers and battering prevention programs: a national survey', *Response* 8: 8–12.
Pleck, J. H. (1981) *The Myth of Masculinity*, Cambridge, Mass.: MIT Press.
Pontin, D. J. T (1988) 'The use of profile similarity indices and the Bem sex role inventory in determining the sex role characterisation of a group of male and female nurses', *Journal of Advanced Nursing* 13: 768–74.
Poole, R. (1993) *The New Sexual Revolution*, London: Hodder & Stoughton.
Pringle, K. (1992) 'Gender politics', *Community Care* (4 March): 16–17.
Ptacek, J. (1988) 'Why do men batter their wives?', in K. Yllo and M. L. Bograd (eds) *Feminist Perspectives on Wife Abuse*, Newbury Park, Cal.: Sage.
Quest, C. (ed.) (1994) *Liberating Women from Modern Feminism*, London: IEA Health and Welfare Unit.
Ramazanoğlu, C. (1989) *Feminism and the Contradictions of Oppression*, London: Routledge.
—— (1992) 'Feminism and liberation', in L. McDowell and R. Pringle (eds) *Defining Women: Social Institutions and Gender Divisions*, Cambridge: Polity Press.
Reid, W. J. (1978) *The Task-centred System*, New York: Columbia University Press.
Reinharz, S. (1992) *Feminist Methods in Social Research*, New York: Oxford University Press.

Renvoize, J. (1993) *Innocence Destroyed: A Study of Child Sexual Abuse*, London: Routledge.

Richardson, D. and Robinson, V. (eds) (1993) *Introducing Women's Studies: Feminist Theory and Practice*, Basingstoke: Macmillan.

Roberts, H. (ed.) (1981) *Doing Feminist Research*, London: Routledge and Kegan Paul.

Rogers, C. R. (1951) *Client-centred Therapy: Its Current Practice, Implications and Theory*, Boston, Mass.: Houghton-Mifflin.

Rose, H. (1986) 'Women's work, women's knowledge', in J. Mitchell and A. Oakley (eds) *What is Feminism?*, Oxford: Blackwell.

Rosenwasser, S. M. and Patterson, W. (1984–85) 'Nontraditional male: men with primary childcare/household responsibilities', *Psychology and Human Development* 1(2): 101–11.

Ross, R., Fabiano, E. and Ross, R. D. (1986) *Reasoning and Rehabilitation: a Handbook for Teaching Cognitive Skills*, Ottawa: Cognitive Centre.

Rubin, L. B. (1983) *Intimate Strangers: What Goes On in Relationships Today, and Why*, New York: Harper and Row.

Russell, G. (1983) *The Changing Role of Fathers*, Milton Keynes: Open University.

—— (1992) *What's He Doing at the Family Centre? The Dilemmas of Men who Care for Children*, London: National Children's Home.

Salter, A. (1988) *Treating Child Sex Offenders and Victims: A Practical Guide*, Newbury Park, Cal.: Sage.

Saunders, D. G. (1988) 'Wife abuse, husband abuse, or mutual combat?', in K. Yllo and M. L. Bograd (eds) *Feminist Perspectives on Wife Abuse*, Newbury Park, Cal.: Sage.

Savage, J. (1987) *Nurses, Gender and Sexuality*, London: Heinemann.

Schechter, S. (1982) *Women and Male Violence: The Visions and Struggles of the Battered Women's Movement*, London: Pluto Press.

Scher, M. Stevens, M. Good, G. and Eichenfield, G. A. (eds) (1987) *Handbook of Counseling and Psychotherapy with Men*, Newbury Park, Cal.: Sage.

Schultz, L. G. (1960) 'The wife assaulter', *Journal of Social Therapy* 6(2): 103–12.

Scottish Office Statistical Bulletin (1992), Edinburgh.

Scottish Office (1992) *Further Education in Scotland*: 1992.

Scottish Prison Service and Social Work Services Group (1989) *Continuity through Co-operation: A National Framework of Policy and Practice Guidance for Social Work in Scottish Penal Establishments: A Consultation Document*, Edinburgh: Scottish Home and Health Department.

Scully, D. (1990) *Understanding Sexual Violence: A Study of Convicted Rapists*, Boston, Mass.: Unwin Hyman.

Seed, P. (1973) *The Expansion of Social Work in Britain*: London: Routledge and Kegan Paul.

Segal, L. (1990a) *Slow Motion: Changing Masculinities, Changing Men*, London: Virago.

—— (1990b) *Straight Sex: The Politics of Pleasure*, London: Virago.

Seidler, V. J. (1989) *Rediscovering Masculinity: Reason, Language and Sexuality*, London: Routledge.

—— (1991a) *Recreating Sexual Politics: Men, Feminism and Politics*, London: Routledge.

—— (ed.) (1991b) *The Achilles Heel Reader: Men, Sexual Politics and Socialism*, London: Routledge.

—— (1991c) 'Men, feminism and patriarchy', in V. J. Seidler (ed.) *The Achilles Heel Reader: Men, Sexual Politics and Socialism*, London: Routledge.

—— (1994) *Unreasonable Men: Masculinity and Social Theory*, London: Routledge.

Sharpe, S. (1994) *Fathers and Daughters*, London: Routledge.

Sheldon, B. (1995) *Cognitive Behaviour Therapy*, London: Routledge.

Silverstein, O. and Rashbaun, B. (1994) *The Courage to Raise Good Men: A Call for Change*, London: Joseph.

Simpson, B., Corlyon, J., McCarthy, P. and Walker, J. (1993) *Post-Divorce Fatherhood*, Newcastle: University of Newcastle upon Tyne.

Sinclair, H. (1989) *Manalive: An Accountable Advocacy Batterer Intervention Program*, Marin County, Cal.: Marin Abused Women's Services.

Sivanandan, A. (1985) 'RAT and the degradation of the black struggle', *Race and Class* 26(4).

Smith, D. E. (1987) *The Everyday World as Problematic: A Feminist Sociology*, Milton Keynes: Open University.

Smith, L. J. F. (1989) *Domestic Violence: An Overview of the Literature*, London: HMSO.

Snodgrass, J. (ed.) (1977) *A Book of Readings for Men Against Sexism*, New York: Times Change Press.

Social Work Services Group and Scottish Home and Health Department (1989) *Continuity through Cooperation: a National Framework of Policy and Practice Guidance of Social Work in Penal Establishments*, Edinburgh: Scottish Office.

Spence, J. (1990) 'Young people, inequality and youth work', in T. Jeffs and M. Smith (eds) *Youth Work and Gender*, London: Macmillan.

Spender, D. (1980) *Man Made Language*, Boston, Mass.: Women's Collective.

—— (1981) *Men's Studies Modified: The Impact of Feminism on the Academic Disciplines*, Oxford: Pergamon.

Stacey, J. (1993) 'Untangling feminist theory', in D. Richardson and V. Robinson (eds) *Introducing Women's Studies: Feminist Theory and Practice*, Basingstoke: Macmillan.

Stanko, E. (1985) *Intimate Intrusions: Women's Experience of Male Violence*, London: Routledge and Kegan Paul.

—— (1994) 'Dancing with denial: researching women and questioning men', in M. Maynard and J. Purvis (eds) *Researching Women's Lives from a Feminist Perspective*, London: Taylor Francis.

Stanley, L. (1982) 'Male needs: the problem of working with gay men', in S. Friedman and E. Sarah (eds) *On the Problem of Men*, London: Women's Press.

—— (1990) *Feminist Praxis: Research, Theory and Epistemology in Feminist Sociology*, London: Routledge.
Stanley, L. and Wise, S. (1983) *Breaking Out: Feminist Consciousness and Feminist Research*, London: Routledge and Kegan Paul.
—— (1993) *Breaking Out Again: Feminist Ontology and Epistemology*, London: Routledge.
Steinmetz, S. K. (1978) 'The battered husband syndrome', *Victimology* 2(3–4): 499–509.
Steinmetz, S. K. and Straus, M. A. (1974) *Violence in the Family*, New York: Dodd, Mead.
Tannen, D. (1992) *You Just Don't Understand: Women and Men in Conversation*, New York: Morrow.
Taylor, B. (1983) *Eve and the New Jerusalem: Socialism and Feminism in the Nineteenth Century*, London: Virago.
Thomas, D. (1993) *Not Guilty: Men: the Case for the Defence*, London: Weidenfeld & Nicolson.
Thompson, N. (1993) *Anti-discriminatory Practice*, Basingstoke: Macmillan.
Thompson, P. (1988) *The Voice of the Past: Oral History*, Oxford: Oxford University Press.
Thorpe, R. and Petruchenia, J. (eds) (1985) *Community Work or Social Change? An Australian Perspective*, London: Routledge & Kegan Paul.
Tolson, A. (1977) *The Limits of Masculinity*, London: Tavistock.
Ungerson, C. (ed.) (1985) *Women and Social Policy: A Reader*, Basingstoke: Macmillan.
—— (1987) *Policy is Personal: Sex, Gender and Informal Care*, London: Tavistock.
Walczak, Y. (1988) *He and She: Men in the Eighties*, London: Routledge.
Walker, A. (1982) *Community Care, the Family, the State and Social Policy* Oxford: Basil Blackwell and Martin Robertson.
Wallerstein, J. and Blakeslee, S. (1989) *Second Chances*, London: Bantam.
Wallerstein, J. and Kelly, J. (1977) 'Divorce counselling: a community service for families in the midst of divorce', *American Journal of Orthopsychiatry* 47(1): 4–22.
—— (1980) *Surviving the Breakup: How Children and Parents Cope with Divorce*, New York: Basic Books.
Walton, R. G. (1975) *Women in Social Work*, London: Routledge and Kegan Paul.
Wasoff, F. (1982) 'Legal protection from wifebeating: the process of domestic assaults by Scottish prosecutors and criminal courts', *International Journal of the Sociology of Law* 10(2): 197–204.
Watkins, S. A., Rueda, M. and Rodriguez, M. (1992) *Feminism for Beginners*, Cambridge: Icon.
Weedon, C. (1987) *Feminist Practice and Poststructuralist Theory*, Oxford: Blackwell.
Williams, C. L. (1989) *Gender Differences at Work*, Berkeley, Cal.: University of California Press.

—— (1993) *Doing 'Women's Work': Men in Nontraditional Occupations*, Newbury Park, Cal.: Sage.

Wilson, A. (1978) *Finding a Voice*, London: Virago.

Wilson, E. (1977) *Women and the Welfare State*, London: Tavistock.

—— (1980) 'Feminism and social work', in R. Bailey and M. Brake (eds) *Radical Social Work and Practices*, London: Edward Arnold.

Wilson, G. (1994) 'Biology, sex roles and work', in C. Quest (ed.) *Liberating Women from Modern Feminism*, London: IEA Health and Welfare Unit.

Wise, S. (1990) 'Becoming a feminist social worker', in L. Stanley and S. Wise (eds) *Feminist Praxis*, London: Routledge.

—— (1992) 'Feminist social work: oppression or liberation?', unpublished lecture to Lothian and Borders Gender Group.

Yllo, K. and Bograd, M. L. (eds) (1988) *Feminist Perspectives on Wife Abuse*, Newbury Park, Cal.: Sage.

Name index

Abbott, P. and Wallace, C. 67
Abramovitz, M. 45, 54
Adams, D. 29, 89, 94, 96, 98
Afshar, H. and Maynard, M. 148
Alcoff, L. and Potter, E. 165
Allen, G. 152
Ambrose, P., Harper, J. and Pemberton, R. 115, 125
Anthias, F. and Yuval-Davis, N. 148
Anzaldua, G. *see* Moraga, C.
Arber, S. and Gilbert, N. 5, 16
Archer, J. 72; and Lloyd, B. B. 52
Arthur, T. A. A. *see* Boreham, N. C.

Bailey, R and Brake, M. 2
Bailey, S. and Cox, P. 55
Baldwin, J. 169
Baker Miller, J. 40, 66
Bancroft, J. 132
Barbaree, H. E., *see* Marshall, W. L.
Barrett, M. 3
Barrett, M.: and McIntosh, M. 148; and Phillips, A. 166
Bart, P. B. and Moran, E. G. 30
Beagley, J. 2
Bell, C. and Roberts, H. 67
Bem, S. L. 67, 71, 72, 82, 86
Bertaux, D. 69
Bhavnani, K. and Coulson, M. 148
Blakeslee, S. *see* Wallerstein, J.
Bly, R. 4, 52, 91, 161, 163, 174
Bograd, M. L. 29, 30

Boreham, N. C. and Arthur, T. A. A. 85
Boston Women's Health Collective 130
Bourne, J. 150
Boushel, M. 62
Bowl, R. 5, 45, 123, 159, 174
Boyle, R. and Curtis, K. 175
Bradshaw, J. 177
Brady, P. 55
Brake, M. *see* Bailey, R.
Brannen, J. 71
Brannon, R. and David, D. S. 175
Brittan, A. 4, 91
Brod, H. 43; and Kaufman, M. xxi
Brook, E. and Davis, A. 2, 114, 181
Brown, W. 148
Brownmiller, S. 52
Bryman, A. 71
Burns, J. and Wright, C. xv, 131
Burns, N., Meredith, C. and Paquette, C. 88
Burton, S. *see* Kelly, L.

Cain, M. 51
Campbell, B. 176, 179
Campbell, J. 169
Canaan, J. E. and Griffin, C. 1
Canton, R. 46
Caplan, P. J. 54
Carby, H.V. 148
Carlen, P. 3
Carli, L. 56, 58

Subject index